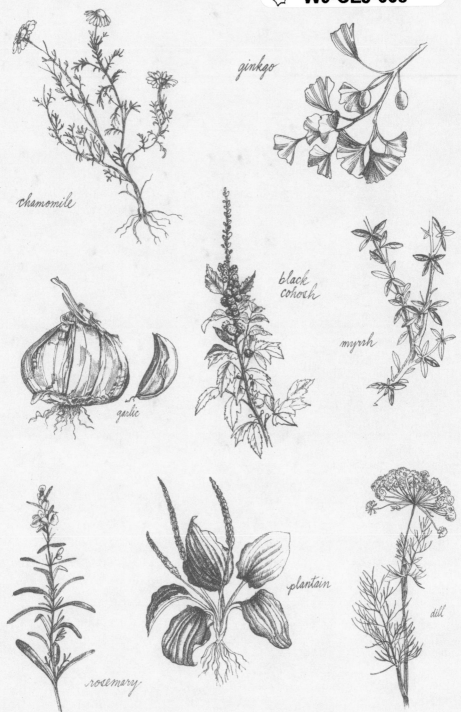

W9-CLJ-668

chamomile

ginkgo

black cohosh

myrrh

garlic

rosemary

plantain

dill

EveryWoman's® Guide to
Natural Home Remedies

Every Woman's® Guide to Natural Home Remedies

....

Sally Freeman

illustrations by
Chris Duke

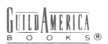

GUILDAMERICA
B O O K S ®

DOUBLEDAY DIRECT, INC.
Garden City, New York

Grateful acknowledgment is made to the following for permission to
reprint their copyrighted material:

Recipe for horehound lozenges on page 116 from *Stalking the Wild
Asparagus* by Euell Gibbons. Copyright © 1962 by Euell Gibbons.
Reprinted by permission of the publisher: Alan C. Hood & Co., Inc.,
P.O. Box 775, Chambersburg, PA 17201.

ISBN: 1-56865-171-6

Although the information and guidance in this book are appropriate
in most cases, and may supplement your physician's advice, it is
recommended that you consult your own physician concerning your
personal medical condition.

Book design by Vertigo Design
Art direction by Nanna Tanier for Doubleday Direct, Inc.

ACKNOWLEDGMENTS

EveryWoman's® Guide to Natural Home Remedies owes much to the contributions of the colleagues, friends, family, consultants, health care organizations and immigrants who helped make it possible.

Foremost, I am indebted to Karen Murgolo, my editor at Guild-America Books®, for her encouragement, enthusiasm, and creative, thoughtful input. Thanks also to Doubleday Direct editors Roz Siegel and Barbara Greenman, who came up with the idea for the book, and to Wendy Lipkind, my literary agent, for bringing me into the project.

Many health care professionals gave generously of their time and knowledge and reviewed chapters. I am grateful to Drs. Maria Arnett, Robin Ashinoff, Dahlia Garza, Debra Guthrie, Howard Liss, Karen Lawson, Melissa Pashcow, and Beth Schorr-Lesnick; to Wendy Iseman, Lisa Long, Betty Kautzman, Hope Martin, and Carole Taylor Schanley. Thanks also to Jimmy Robinson (Jimmy II) for introducing me to Caribbean folk medicine. In particular, my thanks to Ann Darlington, Beth Kruse, Dr. Suzanne Gosselin, and Dr. Lucy Maria Smith for their careful vetting and medical advice.

My thanks to these organizations for information and resources: The Center for Medical Consumers in Manhattan, where much of the library research was done; the Boston Women's Health Collective, the Brooklyn Public Library, Aradia Feminist Health Center, the Vestibular Disorders Association, the American Lung Association, the American Heart Association, the National Dairy Council, the Scleroderma Society, the New England Center for Headache, and The National Women's Health Resource Center.

Finally, my thanks to friends and colleagues who supplied me with information and leads and invaluable support: Olga Melbardis, Ylena Melikian, Sharon Wolf, Susan Cakars, Diana Symonds, Jonathan and Lew Gardner, Father Joe Healey, Elizabeth Lara, Reola Moss, Celia Jaffee, Sharmaine Sacasa, Arlene Kisner, Tony Dread, and Norma Smith; and the immigrant friends in my English as a Second Language classes at New York City Technical College who shared with me the folk medicine of their homelands: Monya Shafir, Bernard Polednik, Justinia Padilla, Oleg Gorodnitskiy, Teresa Moya, Elizabeth Na' Embok, Hector Rodriguez, Yevgeniy Matusevich, Inna

Kopylenko, Diana Vernokova, Viktoriya Griss, Larissa Egorova, Larisa Nisimbaum, Susana Delgado, Mohammed Bensabeur, Edmund Tercy, Teresa Roman Montalvo, Carmen Custodio, Carmen Fleming, Letitia Alonso, and Rosa Serrano.

CONSULTANTS

MARIA F. ARNETT, M.D., Ophthalmologist and Associate Attending Physician at Beth Israel Medical Center in New York City and Associate Attending at New York Eye and Ear Infirmary

ROBIN ASHINOFF, M.D., Chief of Dermatologic and Laser Surgery at New York University Medical Center in New York City

ANN DARLINGTON, M.S., C.N.M., Nurse-Midwife at the Virginia Mason Medical Center's Nurse-Midwifery Service in Seattle, Washington

SUZANNE R. GOSSELIN, B.S.N., D.C., whose practice, Harbor Chiropractic, is in Rockport, Massachusetts

DEBRA S. GUTHRIE, M.D., Attending in Ophthalmology at New York Eye and Ear Infirmary, Beth Israel Medical Center, and New York Downtown Hospital in New York City

WENDY ISEMAN, M.S.W., Communications Director for the American Lung Association of Brooklyn, New York

BETTY KAUTZMANN, P.T., Chief Physical Therapist at the Physical Medicine and Rehabilitation Center in Englewood, New Jersey

BETH KRUSE, C.N.M., of Aradia Feminist Women's Health Center in Seattle, Washington

KAREN LAWSON, M.D., Family Practice Physician currently working in the Emergency Department of Unity Hospital in Minneapolis, Minnesota

HOWARD LISS, M.D., Director of the Physical Medicine and Rehabilitation Center in Englewood, New Jersey; Director of Sports and Musculoskeletal Rehabilitation at Columbia-Presbyterian Medical Center and Assistant Clinical Professor of Rehabilitation Medicine at Columbia University in New York City

LISA LONG, M.P.T., Assistant Chief Physical Therapist at the Physical Medicine and Rehabilitation Center in Englewood, New Jersey

HOPE MARTIN, Certified by the American Center for the Alexander Technique, member of the North American Society of Teachers of the Alexander Technique. Her practice is in New York City

REOLA MOSS, Dental Hygienist at Long Island College Hospital Dental Clinic in Brooklyn, New York

MELISSA S. PASHCOW, M.D., F.A.C.S.,
Associate Attending in the Department
of Otolaryngology at New York Eye
and Ear Infirmary and Clinical
Instructor in Otolaryngology at New
York Medical College, New York City

CAROLE TAYLOR SCHANLEY, Fitness
Instructor and Director of Move It to
Music in Manchester by the Sea,
Massachusetts

BETH SCHORR-LESNICK, M.D., Attending
in Gastroenterology at Beth Israel
Medical Center in New York City, and
Associate Professor of Medicine at
Albert Einstein College of Medicine in
the Bronx, New York

LUCY MARIA SMITH, N.D., Naturopathic
Physician at the Natural Health Clinic
of Bastyr University in Seattle,
Washington

CONTENTS

Introduction

I have given you every herb
bearing seed, which is upon
the face of all the earth, and
every tree, in the which is the
fruit of a tree yielding seed; to
you it shall be for meat.

—GENESIS 1:29

The fruit of the tree is for
man's meat, and the leaves
for man's medicine.

—EZEKIEL 47:12

*h*ome remedies: possibly your mother or
grandmother used them; almost certainly your great-
grandmother did. It may be that you have discovered a
few medical treatments of your own, although you
may not label them as such. For example, what do
you do when you have a sunburn, mosquito bite or
bee sting, a sore throat, charley horse, or hangover?

The various household substances we dab on our skin, the solutions we sip or gargle, the hot bath or shower that banishes stiffness or insomnia—all are home remedies most of us use from time to time, although we may not think to dignify them with that name. Most people learned such strategies for relieving pain, discomfort, or minor ailments as children from their parents, or later, in adulthood, from friends or doctors. The printed sheet of instructions you get from your physician, hospital, or clinic after surgery or treatment for an injury are basically home remedies, although the medical profession refers to them as "self-care."

The use of home remedies is ancient and universal. The foundations of both Eastern and Western healing arts rested upon such folk medicine. In the New World, the original practitioners were the Native Americans who had evolved their own healing techniques using the surrounding woods and fields as a resource, and European settlers, who brought herbal remedies and the seeds for growing them from their native countries. On the early frontier, and later across rural America, where doctors were rare or nonexistent, every family, of necessity, developed a body of knowledge that enabled its members to cope with medical emergencies and chronic illnesses. Through trial and error, people discovered that certain plants could dull pain, bring down a fever, open up the respiratory passages, allay nausea, or bring sleep. For the most part, these remedies had no side effects and were easy to obtain—the reasons people continue to use them today.

African slaves and subsequent immigrants brought home remedies from all corners of the world where the use of medicinal herbs is a recognized and acceptable medical treatment.

The past twenty years or so have seen a renewed interest in folk medicine and herbal remedies. Medical researchers are exploring jungles and rain forests in search of cures for cancer, arthritis, AIDS, and other diseases that all our technologies have so far been unable to cure. Some of our most effective drugs, such as reserpine, digitalis, taxol, and periwinkle, were originally derived from plants.

In the laboratory, popular folk remedies are undergoing scientific scrutiny. Do the natural chemicals in garlic, certain culinary seasonings, or chicken soup actually have medicinal properties? Some of America's leading university research laboratories have confirmed that they do. The newest unit of the National Institutes of Health, the Office of Alternative Therapies, is one of the major research groups investigating folk medicine along with alternative therapies that include yoga, acupuncture, acupressure, vitamin therapy, and Ayurvedic medicine. An increasing number of physicians are using these therapies along with traditional medicine. Because many people these days are experimenting with such techniques at home and passing them on to friends and family, our repertoire of home remedies has greatly expanded to include those once considered exotic.

Manya Shafir, a recent immigrant from Kiev in the former Soviet Union, has been treated with folk medicine since infancy. "Some people say, 'It is not medicine, it's hoodoo,'" Manya relates, "but when they are unable to cope with sickness and weakness, they usually look for folk remedies. The most popular remedy in folk medicine is herbs.

"I grew up in a big family," Manya continues. "My mother mostly treated us with folk medicine. When my children were growing up, I did the same. When a child had an upset stomach, I put warm beets on the stomach. When they caught cold, I made them a tea with chamomile, mint, and honey. When spring came, I gave them rose hips—the best source of vitamin C. Massage and exercise are beautiful remedies to treat the body.

"I think that official medicine shouldn't deny folk medicine. They have to elaborate [complement] each other.

"But all the remedies are only one side of this business," Manya insists. "The other side is the person who prepares the solution. For example, I had a friend in Kiev who was an herbalist. He told me that when he tried to grind his herbs with a machine, it helped less than when he prepared the herbs by hand. He told me, 'In this time when I prepare herbs, I send goodness and best wishes to the sick person.'"

Father Joe Healey, a Maryknoll missionary and author who has lived in Africa for nearly thirty years, and who has written about Africans and their beliefs, noted a similar philosophy among native African healers. "An African herbalist," says Father Healey, "regards gathering the herbs as essential to the healing process. The herbalist looks for propitious signs in the weather and in nature, and goes forth to gather only when he feels an inner harmony. He wouldn't go out gathering herbs when he was angry, for example. The same is true when the healer is grinding the herbs. Herbalists in Africa are good psychologists, able to treat psychosomatic as well as strictly physical illnesses. I have also seen herbalists treat ailments that don't respond to traditional medicine. If you have hepatitis or mononucleosis, there isn't any drug you can take—all you can do is rest and get well. In Tanzania, where I live, they have a white liquid, the color of cream and the texture of maple syrup, that comes from a tree. Different trees have this sap. The Sukuma and Kuria ethnic groups use it to cleanse the system and heal the liver. White sap from a local tree is applied to an open wound to reduce pain. It is also used to reduce the pain of shingles."

Use Common Sense Regarding Home Remedies

On the following pages you will find an array of home remedies from the physicians, midwives, and alternative health practitioners who recommend them, as well as from people all over the world who use them. None of these recommendations are intended to replace the advice of your physician or other health care provider. Although no one is as familiar with your body as you, it is never a good idea to act as your own physician. If your symptoms remain after a few days, seek medical advice. When you do use home remedies, let your doctor know, especially if you are taking other medication. The active ingredients in most home remedies are chemicals—natural ones, to be sure, but chemicals nonetheless. They are capable of causing an allergic reaction in sensitive people, or of interacting adversely with certain chemicals in pharmaceuticals.

It is always a good idea, especially if you have allergies, to test your reaction to an herb by first taking a small quantity accompanied by lots of water. Before you apply them externally, herbs and the oils, lotions, and potions made from them should be first applied to a small area of skin to check for possible irritation. Herbs such as pennyroyal or quinine should not be taken when you are pregnant because they may cause a miscarriage or premature labor. Preparations containing alcohol are also best avoided by pregnant women as well as by anyone recovering from alcohol addiction. Other herbs—for example, comfrey—should not be taken internally. These and other warnings are noted in the text.

How to Use This Book

Remedies are arranged more or less according to the organ system that is affected. The final chapter, "Emergencies," gives first-aid information. Each chapter is introduced by general remarks about the particular body system it is addressing, with advice on keeping it healthy. The information included here is based on research, with the most current information available, as well as interviews with health care professionals and immigrants who have brought their native folk medicines with them to America. Advice from doctors, nurse-midwives, and other practitioners is usually boxed, and the interviewee, with affiliations listed, is introduced near the beginning of the chapter. Later on, the doctor may simply be referred to by name. An appendix lists organizations, newsletters, libraries, and mail order sources for herbs.

In the glossary that follows, you will find descriptions of some of the major alternative therapies that have contributed to our contemporary store of home remedies. You will also find some basic herbal terms used in this book, and instructions for making herbal preparations at home.

Enjoy them in good health!

GLOSSARY

acupressure (also known as Shiatsu) Pressure is applied to points corresponding to sites where acupuncture needles are inserted along the energy network. The fingertips rather than needles are employed to break up energy blocks.

acupuncture An ancient Chinese medical treatment that uses hair-thin needles inserted along the energy network that links all parts of the body. *Qi,* the energy that flows along this network, maintains the body's harmony and balance. Illness can result when this energy is blocked. Perhaps best known for treating addictions and chronic pain, acupuncture is increasingly being incorporated into Western medical practices.

alterative An herb or mineral that gradually alters the course of a disease by improving digestion and elimination.

analgesic An herb or chemical that relieves pain by either blocking sensory nerves or depressing the central nervous system.

antiseptic A substance that kills or inhibits the growth of harmful bacteria. Used to prevent or treat infection on the skin or in the internal organs.

astringent An herb or mineral that causes tissue to contract, arrests mucus or oily secretions, checks bleeding, reduces inflammation, and helps control diarrhea.

Ayurvedic medicine A holistic approach to medicine that was developed in India centuries ago. Uses herbs, diet, exercise, meditation, yoga, and physical therapy to treat imbalances that bring about disease.

carminative An herbal preparation that helps expel intestinal gas and relieve flatulence.

chiropractor A health care professional (D.C.) or Doctor of Chiropractic) who manipulates the spine and, in some states, the extremities, to relieve pain in the skeletal system. Some chiropractors also prescribe vitamins and diets.

compress A cloth or towel soaked in liquid and applied to the skin.

decoction An herbal preparation made by boiling plant seeds, roots, bark, or other tough or woody plant parts in water for ten to thirty minutes. The resulting broth is strained and sipped. Use about one teaspoon dried or 2 teaspoons fresh plant parts to one cup water. (Some herbalists may recommend an ounce plant part to a pint water.)

diaphoretic A substance that stimulates perspiration. Useful in sweating out a cold or bringing down a fever. Works best in a hot drink. Afterward, bundle up and get into bed. Stay warm for at least an hour, ideally for overnight. Be sure to bathe or shower so your skin will not reabsorb toxins released in perspiration.

digestive An herb that aids digestion. Many culinary herbs and herb-based after-dinner liqueurs have this property.

distilling A method of steaming plants so the essence is extracted and concentrated.

diuretic A natural or synthetic chemical that increases the flow of urine, removes fluid from tissues, maintains kidney action, and dilutes urine. When you use diuretics, be sure to replace tissue salts that are excreted in urine. The following formula comes from Dr. Fritz Weiss, author of *Herbal Medicine*: two teaspoons glucose, one teaspoon each peppermint leaves and fennel seeds, $1/2$ teaspoon salt, $1/4$ teaspoon each bicarbonate of soda and potassium chloride, one quart water.

emetic A substance that causes vomiting. Useful in treating some types of poisoning.

emmenagogue An herb or synthetic drug that promotes menstruation. Do not use when pregnant or during heavy menstrual periods.

expectorant An herb or synthetic drug that helps expel mucus from bronchopulmonary passages.

folk medicine A body of medical knowledge discovered primarily by non-physicians, mostly through trial and error, and passed on through generations by oral tradition.

herb Strictly speaking, a woody plant that dies down after flowering. In practice, an herb is just about any plant that is used for culinary or medicinal purposes.

homeopathy Founded by a nineteenth-century German physician, this form of natural healing uses highly diluted herbal or mineral preparations to marshal the body's own defenses against disease. On the premise that "like cures like," tiny doses of substances that would produce the same symptoms in a healthy person are used to stimulate the immune system. (For example, a homeopath might use onion to treat the sniffles.) Some traditional M.D.'s and D.O.'s have incorporated homeopathy into their treatments.

infusion A tea made by steeping plant parts in hot water. The strained liquid can be sipped as a beverage or used as a wash for wounds or skin problems. Unless the instructions tell you otherwise, when a home remedy calls for an herbal infusion, use one teaspoon dry or two teaspoons fresh leaves to one cup boiling water. Steep—do not boil—for ten minutes, and sip slowly—by the teaspoonful is best.

naturopathy A system of holistic medicine developed in the nineteenth century. Based on the premise that the body is capable of healing itself once the proper conditions are provided, naturopathy employs herbs, homeopathy, nutrition, fasting, physiotherapy, and exercise. Practitioners receive four years of postgraduate medical training and do not perform surgery or prescribe pharmaceuticals.

osteopathy A system of medicine founded by A. T. Still in 1864 that includes all aspects of allopathic medicine and surgery, as well as a holistic philosophy and manipulative medicine skills. Minimum requirement for practice as a D.O. is essentially the same as for M.D.'s: four years of medical school and one year of internship. M.D.'s and D.O.'s have equal practice rights in all 50 states.

physiatry A branch of medicine that deals with musculoskeletal injuries and rehabilitation through exercise, physiotherapy, and other techniques.

poultice A mass of heated herbs laid directly on the skin. If the herbs are fresh, crush or pound them to release their healing properties; if they are dried, soak them for about ten minutes in a little hot water. Cover the herbs with a warm, moist cloth that is kept warm by frequent dipping in hot water. Mustard, pepper, garlic, and other irritating substances should not be laid directly on the skin—wrap them in a cloth first and check frequently to make sure the skin isn't blistered.

reflexology A form of natural healing where practitioners manipulate and massage certain areas on the feet that correspond to specific organs.

sedative A botanical or synthetic drug that soothes the nerves.

sitz bath A shallow bath that comes no higher than your navel. You can use anything big enough to sit in, from a basin to a bathtub.

tincture A preparation made by steeping herbs in alcohol. Alcohol extracts properties of herbs that are not water-soluble; it is also a preservative that allows you to store an herb for a relatively long time. If you cannot take alcohol, you can buy or make tinctures based on cider vinegar. To make a tincture, add one-quarter to one ounce powdered herb to eight to ten ounces tasteless spirits such as vodka. Depending on the proof of the alcohol, add enough water to make a 50 percent solution. Seal the bottle and let it stand for two weeks, shaking it once or twice a day. Strain and add a few drops to a teaspoonful to a glass of water and take orally. You can also take tinctures undiluted.

tonic Foods and herbs that strengthen and invigorate certain organs or the entire system.

The Reproductive System:

From Breast-feeding to Vaginitis

O nce you reach sexual maturity, your sense of physical and emotional well-being is largely determined by the complex relationship between your nervous system and the hormones produced by your ovaries, adrenals, and pituitary gland. During your reproductive years, your menstrual cycle is influenced by the fluctuating balance between your estrogen and progesterone levels, both necessary for establishing and maintaining a healthy pregnancy and for protecting your bones and heart.

Exercise and a healthy diet are crucially important. The essential nutrients for women are calcium and vitamin E, the former to ensure strong bones for you and your offspring, the latter for healthy reproductive organs, efficient use of oxygen, and a strong cardiovascular system.

Breast-feeding

There is much to be said for a mode of baby feeding that demands no sterilizing before, or warming after, and requires only a portable container that never gets mislaid. Even more important, breast milk, especially colostrum, the sticky yellow fluid secreted by the mammary glands for a day or two before the mature breast milk comes in, helps protect infants from infections, intestinal disorders, and respiratory disease. Yet another benefit is that nursing your baby helps shrink your uterus to its normal size, thus reducing the size of the placental site and the amount of placental bleeding. Although hormone levels and uterine contractions during lactation make pregnancy less likely, don't count on nursing as your means of contraception: women do get pregnant while breast-feeding.

Insufficient Milk

Sometimes a lactating mother's mammary glands don't produce much milk, or the supply is not adequate to baby's demand. It may take a few days to establish a good flow, particularly if you are nursing your first baby. Frequent sucking stimulates your mammary glands to secrete more milk. Drinking a lot of fluid, including daily a quart of milk, helps ensure this.

The amount of rest and relaxation you get is another important factor. If you are tired and harried, as so many women are these days, you may have breast-feeding problems. Early evening is the time when you are most likely to run out of milk because of exhaustion. An afternoon nap, or at least a rest, helps you avoid this.

Emotional support is an essential element of your success. LaLeche League has been providing information and support to nursing mothers for decades. See your phone book for the chapter nearest you.

If home remedies don't work for you, see your health care provider —there could be a hormonal or glandular problem.

Ann Darlington (C.N.M., M.S., A.R.N.P.), Nurse-Midwife at the Virginia Mason Medical Center's Nurse-Midwifery Service in Seattle, Washington, has this advice about increasing milk production:

Beer and stout, traditional remedies, are effective because of the hops, which stimulate milk. But remember that everything you take into your body will enter your milk—that includes the alcohol as well as the hops. Your best strategy, known as the twenty-four-hour cure, is to go to bed for twenty-four hours. During this time, everyone should cater to you while you do nothing but sleep, nurse, and drink lots of fluid, including a quart of milk. The increased sucking and emptying of your breasts increases the milk supply over the next one to three days.

Drink at least a quart of fluid daily, and take in at least 1,500 milligrams of calcium. Dairy products are your richest source, but the current practice of adding hormones and antibiotics to milk has some women worried about the effect on their children and themselves. Some dairy producers ensure purity. Their milk is sold in food co-ops, health food stores, and some supermarkets. Alternate calcium sources include canned sardines and salmon with bones, chicken stock made with bones, soy or nut milks, dried beans, tofu, and leafy greens (except for spinach, turnip greens, and other greens high in oxalic acid, which leaches calcium from the bones).

Caffeine accelerates calcium loss from your bones, so drink caffeinated coffee, tea, cocoa and soft drinks sparingly.

Calcium Sources
(according to the National Dairy Council)

1 cup skim milk = 302 mg

1 ounce cheddar cheese = 204 mg

3 ounces canned sardines with bones = 372 mg

3 ounces canned salmon with bones = 167 mg

1 cup cooked dried beans = 90 mg

4 ounces tofu, processed with calcium sulfate = 145 mg

$^{1}/_{2}$ cup cooked collard greens = 149 mg

Herbal and Folk Remedies

FENNEL SEEDS boiled in barley milk, and anise, dill, caraway, or coriander seeds boiled in water are all used in folk medicine, both for stimulating mother's milk and for relieving baby's colic. In Belize, nursing mothers eat plantains and drink coconut milk to stimulate lactation. Apple cider, which is said to maintain a healthy pH level in the body, helps some women increase their milk supply.

Sore Nipples

First-time mothers and fair-skinned women are the most likely to have tender, raw nipples.

Avoiding and coping with sore nipples
Advice from nurse-midwife Ann Darlington:

- A baby's gums are really bones covered by thin mucous membrane, and they can hurt if they close on your nipple. Teach your baby to take as much of the entire areola as possible. Make sure there is a good attachment by taking the nipple out of the baby's mouth if the infant is not latched on well. (First break the suction by putting your finger in the baby's mouth.)

- The easiest way to deal with sore nipples is to express a few drops of colostrum or breast milk and rub it on your nipples after each feeding and between feedings if possible—it's remarkably healing.

- The tannic acid in black tea can heal and toughen your nipples. Moisten a tea bag and use it as a compress against your nipples for ten minutes, then air-dry your nipple for another ten minutes.

Beth Kruse (C.N.M., A.R.N.P.) of Aradia Feminist Women's Health Center in Seattle advises:

Soaps, salves, and creams are not recommended. It is best to go braless as much as possible, expose your nipples to sun and air, gradually build up your baby's time on each breast, and use natural vitamin E oil after you air-dry your nipples following each feeding. Ice packs afterward help, too.

Herbal and Folk Remedies

ALOE VERA, a panacea for skin injuries and disorders, is the choice of women who live in the tropics. In Belize, nursing women relieve sore nipples with cocoa butter or coconut oil. Squaw vine berries mixed with cream or oil are also said to be effective.

Breast Infection

Pain, swelling, redness, tenderness, and sometimes heat or fever can be signs of a breast infection, especially if you are nursing. It is caused by various bacteria, and if home remedies are not effective, it is usually treated by antibiotics. You can almost always continue to breast-feed while on carefully selected antibiotics. If home remedies don't clear up the problem in a day or two, see a doctor immediately.

Engorgement of your breast and stagnation of milk in the ducts can exacerbate infection. Frequent emptying of your breasts, high fluid intake, and rest are critical.

Acetaminophen is safe to take for bringing down a fever and relieving overall aches and pains.

Herbal and Folk Remedies

TRY HERBAL compresses of goldenseal or echinacea (2 teaspoons powdered herb to one cup boiling water) at least three times a day. Apply a hot compress for three minutes followed by a cold compress for thirty seconds. For antimicrobial and immune-stimulating effects, take echinacea internally in capsule form or tea.

Childbirth

Latent, or False, Labor

Although your uterus contracts throughout pregnancy, at about the time you expect to give birth, or shortly before, you may experience contractions that feel like labor. However, these contractions, unlike those of true labor, do not increase in intensity and length, nor is the time between them shortened. If you feel these contractions before your thirty-eighth week of pregnancy, be sure to contact your prenatal care provider immediately.

Awaiting real labor
Nurse-midwife Ann Darlington offers this advice:

- Latent labor can last as long as two days before the onset of the contractions that bring about the cervical changes leading to childbirth. If this happens, talk to your health care provider.

- A supportive environment is very important. Arrange to have your mate or a close friend with you as you await the onset of true labor.

- Sleep as much as you can, if only between contractions, so you will have as much energy as possible when you finally give birth. Warm baths help you relax.

- Sometimes dehydration or hyperglycemia are the culprits behind ineffective contractions. Take in fluids and carbohydrates and other easily digested foods.

- If, despite your efforts to relax and rest, the ineffective contractions continue, you may want to speed up the process. Massage one breast until you have a contraction. If your body doesn't respond, massage the other breast, or both together. As soon as you get a contraction, stop the massage until the contraction ends. Discontinue the massage altogether if your contractions last longer than one minute, or if they are closer together than three minutes from the beginning of one to the beginning of the next. This is to avoid stressing the baby by diminished blood flow to and through the placenta.

- You can also stimulate real labor by walking around or making love. **Warning:** To avoid the risk of infection or trauma, do not engage in sex if your waters have broken or there is bleeding.

Herbal and Folk Remedies

FOR CENTURIES, folk medicine has used herbs to excite uterine contractions. During the Middle Ages, midwives used ergot, a rust that grows on rye and barley; Amerindians and probably Colonial midwives used blue cohosh root. Juniper berries, an ingredient in gin, and various purgatives have also been used at different phases of pregnancy to bring on either labor or an abortion. Needless to say, you should not try any of these without first consulting your health care provider.

Perineal Tears

To avoid tearing the perineum—the tissue that connects your anus and vagina—when the baby's head emerges during childbirth, a doctor may make an incision. Some advocates of unmedicated childbirth try to circumvent this minor surgery, known as an episiotomy, by various strategies explained below. Nurse-midwife Beth Kruse of Seattle's Aradia notes that whether or not you will have perineal tearing has much to do with the skill and patience of your birth attendant.

Avoiding perineal tears
Nurse-midwife Ann Darlington offers this advice:

- Whether or not you will need an episiotomy to avoid tearing when your baby is born depends on how elastic your perineum is. Genetics are the determining factor, but if you have birthed before, this area will be more elastic.

- Kegel exercises, which tone the muscles of your pelvic floor, are especially important during pregnancy because they prepare you for giving birth. These exercises consist of contracting and releasing the muscles surrounding your vagina and anus—

see SEX AND ORGASM (page 35) for details.

- To strengthen your thighs and open up your pelvic area, giving more room to the developing fetus, squat for a few seconds at a time with your knees out and your heels down, either in a freestanding position or leaning against a wall.

- The trauma of labor tightens your perineum. Massage helps relax the area and may shorten labor if you have learned to relax rather than tighten.

- Unfortunately, research hoping to show that perineal massage would reduce the incidence of tearing or the rare need for episiotomy has not supported that theory.

- To heal postdelivery tears and stitches, use ice packs at hourly intervals for the first twelve hours, then sitz baths until the area is healed. Soak daily in hip-deep water, using a portable showerhead (if available) to make a Jacuzzi—the flowing water helps clean up cellular debris and stimulate circulation. If the tears are severe, take three or four sitz baths a day. It is okay to take a nice deep soak in the tub; just don't wash your body and then soak in the dirty water.

- Anemia makes it harder to heal a severe tear, so be sure to get a lot of rest if you have this problem to enhance healing and increase stamina. You may also need postpartum iron supplements.

Herbal and Folk Remedies

RUBBING VITAMIN E oil on your perineum for a month or two before you expect to give birth aids elasticity.

IF AN episiotomy is necessary, some birthing centers use a poultice of comfrey leaves to speed healing. To make a poultice, spread fresh, bruised leaves or dry leaves softened by boiling water on a sterile cloth or cheesecloth and leave it on the area for fifteen to twenty minutes. Repeat three times daily. Allantoin, a cell-proliferant in comfrey, speeds healing by rapidly replacing damaged skin cells with new ones.

Stretch Marks

These pearly scars are left when your skin resumes its original shape after it has been stretched. Weight gain and loss can leave stretch marks on your breasts, thighs, and sometimes upper arms; pregnancy often leaves stretch marks on the abdomen. The more excess weight you gain, the more stretch marks you will have.

Nurse-midwife Ann Darlington on stretch marks:

Whether or not you have stretch marks depends on your genes, which determine your body's design and how much the elastin fibers stretch. Nothing has been shown to really work except maybe retin A, which can cause birth defects if taken when you're pregnant. Any effect of retin A on stretch mark reduction disappears as soon as you discontinue its use, anyway. Try to think of these scars as a tribute to your body's ability to change dramatically in pregnancy, and wear them with pride as one who has birthed.

Herbal and Folk Remedies

A UNIVERSAL stretch mark preventative is to rub olive oil on your abdomen throughout pregnancy and until your belly resumes its natural size. Vitamin E oil, said to prevent scarring, can be used in the same way.

ALOE VERA is a folk remedy used in the tropics for all sorts of skin problems, including scarring.

Swelling of Feet and Legs

During the latter months of pregnancy your legs, ankles, and feet may swell, especially during hot weather. Some swelling during pregnancy is inevitable because your body stores up extra fluid against the blood loss you will experience at delivery. However, you should check with your health care provider, because swollen extremities or sudden facial swelling can be a sign of induced hypertension, preeclampsia, or toxemia.

Sodium causes water retention, so keep intake at a minimum. It is a good idea to put away your salt shaker from the time you learn you are pregnant until you finish breast-feeding. And watch out for hidden sodium in canned and prepared foods, condiments, soy and hot sauces, pickled foods, and commercial salad dressings.

Water is an excellent diuretic. It helps shift water out of your tissues, back into your bloodstream and ultimately your kidneys and bladder. Thus, you eliminate more water than you take in. (See also information on water immersion under VARICOSE VEINS, page 90.) Water also dilutes sodium, especially if you add lemon juice.

Varicose Veins

See Chapter Four, "The Cardiovascular System," pages 90–91.

Conception

To learn when you are fertile, advises nurse-midwife Ann Darlington, study your personal menstrual cycle. Most women ovulate, and thus are fertile, about two weeks before they menstruate.

Basal body temperature is higher just before ovulation. Take your temperature just before you get up in the morning, and keep a daily record for a few months.

At ovulation, your body is prepared to welcome sperm: your cervix is slightly open, you are more interested in sex, and your mucus is thin and wet so the sperm can swim easily toward your womb. Just before you ovulate, when estrogen is high, your mucus is fertile, thin, stretchy, and clear. When you are not ovulating, your mucus is thick and ropy, making it hard for the sperm to swim through. Although fluctuations in mucus consistency is not readily apparent by casual observation, women who have regularly examined their vaginal mucus can detect differences in sight, touch, and even taste.

Genetic researcher Margaret Hightower explains that regularly examining vaginal mucus is an ancient method of determining fertility cycles that was practiced by Native Americans. Cycles can vary from one month to another, and even a consistent cycle can vary in any one month for emotional, physical, or dietary reasons. The advantage of this method is that it evaluates each cycle individually.

If the normal 4.5 pH of your vagina is altered by douching, it can interfere with conception. Douching is rarely necessary—our bodies cleanse themselves.

A well-balanced diet helps you establish and maintain a healthy pregnancy. Wheat germ oil, raw wheat germ, and alfalfa are excellent sources of vitamin E, essential to the reproductive functioning of both sexes. Alfalfa is also rich in vitamin K, which helps prevent miscarriage.

Stress depletes folic acid, which helps prevent birth defects. Lettuce, whole grains, nuts, brewer's yeast, and liver are good sources of this B vitamin. Include plentiful amounts in your diet for a few months before trying to conceive.

Herbal and Folk Remedies

Increasing the possibility of conception—
Advice from Dr. Lucy Maria Smith, M.D., a naturopathic physician
at the Natural Health Clinic of Bastyr University in Seattle:

- I often prescribe MCHU tincture, an old naturopathic midwife's tonic used to prepare the body for pregnancy. Sometimes called "Mother's Cordial," the tincture is also taken in the last month to ensure a successful delivery. It is composed of four herbs: squaw vine, squawroot, blue cohosh, and cramp bark.

- Caffeine depletes B vitamins and prostaglandins essential for hormone balance, so you would be wise to cut down or eliminate its use.

- Raising your progesterone level before pregnancy may be helpful, especially if you have a history of miscarriages. The herbs sarsaparilla, Mexican yam, and licorice are good sources. Natural progesterone cream is also sold in some health food stores. See PREMENSTRUAL SYNDROME (pages 30–32) for details. **Don't take any of these herbs after you are pregnant.**

DANDELION ROOT coffee is said to reduce the craving for caffeine and is high in iron and vitamins.

TEA MADE from raspberry leaves or black haw (a botanical relative of the cranberry, available in herbal outlets), taken several times a day, a mouthful at a time, is used in folk medicine to help prevent miscarriages.

Contraception

By determining your fertility cycle (see the preceding section, CONCEPTION) you can decide when to abstain from sex or to use short-term birth control methods.

Barrier contraceptives such as cervical caps, diaphragms, and condoms work for many women, but they are not foolproof. According to 1993 statistics published by the Guttmacher Institute, 18 percent of women experience pregnancy in the first year of average (i.e., not perfect) use of the cervical cap or diaphragm; 16 percent of women get pregnant in the first year of average condom use. If no contraceptive method is used, the pregnancy rate is 85 percent. In order to be effective, these barrier methods must be used correctly and every time you have intercourse (consult your health care provider for instructions). Condoms protect against sexually transmitted diseases as well as pregnancy. If you need additional lubrication, avoid petroleum jelly, which degrades the latex in barrier contraceptives.

Herbal and Folk Remedies

THE FOLK remedies described here are included mainly for historical interest. How useful at preventing conception they prove to be depends on luck, genetics, and fertility.

IN SIBERIA, women abstain from intercourse two or three days before ovulation; at other times they insert a slice of lemon in the vagina twenty minutes before making love. An ancient method of birth control was similar: In countries where it grew, a half lemon, hollowed out, was used like a diaphragm or cervical cap.

APPALACHIAN WOMEN drink a teaspoonful of Queen Anne's lace seeds in a glass of water immediately after sex. In parts of India, women chew the seeds. A chemical in the seeds inhibits production of progesterone, necessary for establishing pregnancy.

IN LABORATORY studies, eating pomegranate seeds has been shown to reduce fertility.

EATING THE leaves and seeds of acacia gum, another folk contraceptive, prevented pregnancy in laboratory rats.

TEA MADE with the herb motherwort has been used by Chinese women as a contraceptive for two thousand years.

Fibrocystic Breasts/ Uterine Fibroids

Fibroids are benign tumors that grow on the inner, center, or outer wall of the uterus. Their growth is linked with estrogen; they usually shrink and may even disappear after menopause. Excessive caffeine intake is thought to be a contributing factor. Sometimes they cause heavy bleeding or pain. Although hysterectomies were formerly the remedy of choice for most doctors, they are a drastic and usually unnecessary procedure. Because hysterectomy causes early menopause, many doctors nowadays tend to leave the fibroids alone unless excessive bleeding, pain, interference with other organs, or other complications undermine the health of the patient. Also, if you plan to get pregnant, your doctor may advise you to have the fibroids removed, especially if they are on the inner uterine walls.

Fibrocystic breasts are often lumpy and sometimes tender. This, too, is a benign condition. The only known risk is that these cysts may make other lesions difficult to detect. Fibroids or fibrocystic breasts should be checked out by your doctor.

Avoiding or reducing fibrocystic breasts or uterine fibroids
Naturopathic physician Dr. Lucy Smith has these suggestions:

- Dairy products, eggs, red meat, and other foods that promote mucus can cause tumors and cysts. They should be avoided, along with coffee (which studies show is linked with fibrous growth), white flour, refined foods, poultry, sugar, tea, cola drinks, chocolate, and alcohol.

- Substitute unsaturated oils for saturated fats and margarine.

- Increase your intake of fresh fruits and vegetables, nuts, seeds, whole grains, and legumes.

- Take in lots of water, beta carotene, calcium, zinc, magnesium, iodine, selenium, and vitamins B, C, and E.

- Natural progesterone, available in many health food stores as a cream derived from Mexican yams or soybeans, is proving helpful for many female reproductive disorders, including fibrous breasts. Apply $1/8$ to $1/4$ teaspoon directly to your breasts.

Menopause

Menopause can occur anytime between the ages of forty-five and sixty, but most women experience it around age fifty-two. Some women have a cluster of symptoms; others have only the absence of menstrual periods. Much depends upon individual physiology and the family genes; the rest has to do with how well a woman takes care of herself, both physically and emotionally. For some, the staging area of menopause is primarily the mind rather than the body. Our sense of well-being, here as elsewhere, depends on how we see ourselves, and, inevitably, the way society views older women.

Some women have menopausal symptoms for years before their periods cease. The drop in estrogen and progesterone levels is gradual and actually begins when a woman reaches her twenties. Even after menopause, the ovaries continue to produce some estrogen. Fleshy women have higher levels because fatty tissue converts other substances to estrone, a type of estrogen usually formed by conversion of estradiol, the form of estrogen manufactured by the ovaries.

Beth Kruse of Aradia notes that many menopausal symptoms may not be related to estrogen levels at all but to the increase in follicle-stimulating hormone from the pituitary gland, which interferes with the brain's production of endorphins and corticosteroids. She adds that there is often no measurable decline in estrogen until about six months without a menstrual period, often years after the first menopausal symptoms.

Because estrogen is thought to protect women from heart disease, osteoporosis, and less serious problems such as hot flashes, the synthetic hormone is routinely prescribed. Studies have shown that taking synthetic estrogen leads to an increased risk of endometrial and breast cancers, circulatory disorders, stroke, fibroid tumors, and fibrocystic breasts. Don't take this hormone if you smoke or carry extra weight, especially if the estrogen is unopposed by progesterone.

Symptoms that are associated particularly with menopause are discussed below. Others, such as weight gain, insomnia, osteoporosis, and constipation, are treated in the appropriate sections (see index).

Herbal and Folk Remedies

CERTAIN HERBS contain phytoestrogens, hormone-like compounds that are chemically similar to estrogen. These include the Chinese herbs ginseng, don quai (Chinese angelica), and fo-ti (Ho Shou Wu); also licorice, red clover, black cohosh, and star root (*Aletris farinosa*).

A 1990 REPORT in *The British Medical Journal* stated that women increased their estrogen level when they ate foods that raised the estrogen level in farm animals. According to Claude L. Hughes, a gynecologist with Duke University, these foods include alfalfa, anise, apples, barley, carrots, cherries, clover, coffee, fennel, garlic, green beans, hops, licorice, oats, parsley, peas, pomegranates, potatoes, red beans, rice, rye, sage, sesame seeds, soybeans and sprouts, wheat, and yeast.

TO REDUCE the risk of cancer, estrogen in any form should always be taken with some form of progesterone for hormonal balance. Dr. John Lee, a well known holistic physician, and expert on natural progesterone who practices in California, recommends a daily dose of natural progesterone from Mexican yam or soybeans.

Coping with menopause
Advice from naturopathic physician Dr. Lucy Smith:

In addition to vitamin E, exercise, foods rich in calcium and vitamin D, and emotional support, use plant estrogens for menopause. One of the most convenient forms of plant estrogens I often recommend a formula called Ostaderm 118 by Bezweken of Portland, Oregon. The preparation contains plant progesterones and plant estrogens and is formulated as a cream. Rub $1/4$ teaspoon into the skin each day for three weeks of each month, then discontinue use for one week of the month. Similar plant estrogen creams are sold in health food stores.

Hot Flashes

The most notorious menopausal symptom, hot flashes, consist of a sudden sensation of warmth, typically lasting from fifteen seconds to a minute, sometimes accompanied by a tingling sensation and/or reddening of the skin. In some feminist circles they are known as "power surges." Stress, caffeine, alcohol, spicy foods, and hot drinks can trigger a hot flash. Women who are prone to flashes find it helpful to dress in layers (preferably cotton) that can be rapidly peeled off at the onset of a hot flash.

Dr. Lucy Smith explains that arteries have tiny muscle fibers in the walls that allow them to constrict in response to various stimuli. In hot flashes, it seems that the changing hormonal milieu causes fluctuations in the artery's diameter. Dilation causes the blood flow to the surface of your skin that you perceive as a hot flash. Vitamin E stabilizes your blood vessels so they don't vary as much in response to the hormones.

Sources for vitamin E include wheat germ and wheat germ oil, corn, safflower, sesame, soy, and peanut oils, seeds, peanuts, Brazil nuts, hazelnuts, lamb, liver, herring, mackerel, kale, cucumber, peas, asparagus, brown rice, and millet.

Some women reduce the frequency and severity of hot flashes by taking 400 to 1,600 international units (IUs) of vitamin E after a meal containing fat. A combination of vitamin E, ginseng, and vitamin C can also be helpful. Selenium assists vitamin E in its functions. Food sources include brewer's yeast, garlic, liver, tuna fish, whole grains, and eggs. If you prefer supplements, take 25 milligrams of selenium with each 200 IUs of vitamin E. Some products combine the two. **Note:** If you have diabetes, high blood pressure, a rheumatic heart condition or take digitalis, consult your physician before taking vitamin E supplements.

Fifty to 200 milligrams of vitamin B6, which is depleted at menopause, may also be helpful in controlling hot flashes. Do not take higher doses without consulting your doctor first.

Hot flash recipes from the Santa Fe Health Education Project:

- Two tablespoons alfalfa seeds steeped for ten minutes in boiling water. Take with lemon three times a day.

- One ounce wild marjoram in one pint hot—but not boiling—water. Allow the mixture to cool, then strain and add a cup of port wine. Take one tablespoonful three times a day before meals.

- Two parts each motherwort and red sage to one part each tansy, pennyroyal, and skullcap. Take one teaspoonful (steeped for ten minutes in boiling water, then cooled to lukewarm) three times a day before meals.

Herbal and Folk Remedies

AT THE onset of a hot flash, drink cold water or juice or chew the root of don quai (Chinese angelica), a source of phytoestrogen.

SOAK IN a bathtub filled with warm water and a cup of Epsom salts until the bathwater cools. The salts are a good source of magnesium, which may be depleted at menopause.

HERBS THAT have been used for hot flashes include cramp bark, goldenseal, red raspberry leaves, spearmint, red clover, wormseed, fennel, and gotu kola. Sarsaparilla, don quai, black cohosh, blue cohosh, unicorn and false unicorn roots, wild yam root, red clover, and panax ginseng contain plant hormones.

A TONIC many women have found helpful is ½ teaspoon each motherwort, spearmint, red clover, squaw vine, don quai, gotu kola, licorice, black cohosh, and sarsaparilla steeped in one cup boiling water for ten minutes. To spare yourself the bother of daily mixing, make up large batches of the tea and refrigerate.

DR. JOHN LEE recommends natural progesterone taken every fifteen minutes when you experience hot flashes.

Night Sweats

Some women experience hot flashes accompanied by perspiration; other women have sweats but no flashes. In either case, heavy sweating is particularly troublesome when it occurs at night, sometimes even soaking the bedclothes.

As with other menopausal symptoms, most women find that regular exercise and sensible nutrition are the best preventatives. Extra calcium and vitamin E may also bring relief.

At bedtime, drink one teaspoon dried sage steeped for ten minutes in one cup boiling water. Sage suppresses perspiration and also contains natural estrogen.

Vaginal Dryness

Vaginal dryness can be caused by many conditions, including emotional stress, surgery, and certain medications. Some women experience postpartum dryness, especially if they are breast-feeding, but most dryness results from the estrogen decline after menopause.

The texture of aloe vera gel is similar to that of vaginal fluids. Mix in a capsule of vitamin E oil and use the mixture as a lubricant. Astroglide and other over-the-counter preparations are also good. Petroleum jelly is not recommended—it is not water-soluble and it degrades the latex in condoms, diaphragms, and cervical caps.

Be sure to include some oil in your diet. How much varies with the individual; two to three tablespoons is usually sufficient.

Supplements of natural estrogen or progesterone, or using progesterone cream for lubrication may be helpful, but these should be prescribed by a naturopathic physician or other health care professional familiar with their properties.

Regular sexual activity, with or without a partner, helps keep your vagina healthy and moist.

Menstruation

The hormones estrogen and progesterone trigger key events in your menstrual cycle. The former is actually a group of hormones produced by your reproductive glands and adrenal organs. It thickens the lining of your uterus and signals your ovary to release the egg. Progesterone prepares your uterine lining to receive the egg. Once the egg is fertilized, progesterone protects your fetus from miscarriage and prepares your mammary glands to produce milk. If the egg is not fertilized, progesterone declines and your uterine lining is sloughed off in menstruation.

Menstrual Cramps

Many women, particularly those who have not borne a child, have experienced painful uterine contractions that can radiate from the abdomen to the back or thighs, and may be accompanied by nausea, diarrhea, sweating, and/or fainting. Possible causes include the release of excess prostaglandin hormones, which cause the uterus to contract painfully; fibroids; polyps; stress; endometriosis; ovarian cysts; cervical stenosis; IUDs; and infection.

Regular vigorous exercise, which stimulates painkiller endorphins and improves pelvic circulation, combined with a diet low in fats, sugar, salt, and dairy products, may help prevent or correct the problem over time.

Increased intake of certain nutrients may help: B complex vitamins, especially B6, vitamin E, beta carotene, zinc, and magnesium. The latter relaxes your muscles—and the uterus is a large muscular organ. To be sure you get enough of these vitamins and minerals, eat lots of whole grains, especially wheat germ; nuts; leafy greens and yellow vegetables; and fruits. The drop in blood calcium level that occurs about a week before you menstruate can cause cramping of your uterine wall when flow begins, so take extra calcium at this time.

A soak in a hot bath will help relieve muscle tension. Try adding a cup or so of Epsom salts, a rich source of magnesium. Alternating hot and cold packs may also bring relief.

Practicing yoga improves pelvic and glandular circulation. The Cobra is possibly the best-known posture for toning the pelvic organs and relieving cramps. Lie facedown on the floor with some padding under you, legs together, arms above your head. Slowly, to a count of ten, lift your head, then your shoulders and chest, supporting the weight of your torso on your outstretched hands. Take ten deep breaths, then slowly lower your upper torso to a count of ten.

Dr. Lucy Smith recommends this posture, which should be held for one to five minutes

Lie on your back with your legs outstretched, small of your back flattened against the floor. Press the fingers of both hands firmly but sensitively downward just above your pubic hairline, drawing the skin of your abdomen towards your navel.

Herbal and Folk Remedies

APPLY ⅛ to ¼ teaspoon natural progesterone cream to your pelvic area. The cream, derived from Mexican yams, is available in some health food stores.

IN CHINA, women avoid cramps by refraining from both iced and very hot drinks during their periods.

IN THE Caribbean, women drink bitters, a solution of alcohol and herbs. In America, bitters are used to flavor cocktails and are sold in some supermarkets.

IN RUSSIA, women dress in warm clothes, drink chamomile tea, apply a heating pad to the painful area, or place a hot water bottle between their legs.

TINCTURE OF cramp bark, sold in health food stores, is very effective for some women. Other herbal tinctures or teas that help ease cramps are chamomile, feverfew, black haw bark, pasqueflower, black cohosh root, Jamaica dogwood bark, squaw vine, white willow, ginger, angelica, wild yam, mother-of-thyme, or a mixture of spearmint, peppermint, and lemon balm. Juniper berries also ease cramps.

ALCOHOL IS both a painkiller and a blood thinner. For this reason, a few doctors recommend a shot or two of gin containing juniper berries.

Delayed Menstruation

Although the average menstrual cycle is twenty-eight days, it can "normally" range from twenty-five to thirty-five days, varying with the individual, and sometimes fluctuating from month to month. To determine your cycle, keep a record of your periods (menses) for a few months. Tardy or irregular menstruation has a variety of causes, including pregnancy and menopause. If you live in a household with other menstruating females, you may note that your cycles gradually alter so they coincide. Poor nutrition, anemia, stress, and overly strenuous exercise can result in delayed or even skipped periods, but so can more serious problems, including hormonal imbalances and tumors, so see your health care provider before you undertake home remedies.

Adequate rest, a well-balanced diet rich in iron, drinking a quart or two of water daily, and sensible exercise should help keep your reproductive system healthy. Daily yoga practice is great for hormonal balance, reproductive toning, and bringing your periods into the twenty-eight-day cycle.

Herbal and Folk Remedies

HERBS THAT were included in the turn-of-the-century U.S. Pharmacopoeia (which lists official natural and synthetic drugs currently in use) were fresh aloe vera juice, taken internally to improve pelvic circulation, and black haw, which can improve flow by relieving pain and irritation.

THE HERB squaw vine, known as the "female regulator," and black cohosh are prescribed by homeopaths for both suppressed and excessive menstruation. Both these herbs, as well as black haw, are ingredients in the Lydia Pinkham herbal compound, which has been used for "female complaints" for decades and is still sold today.

HOT BATHS and hot drinks have been used for centuries to "bring down the courses," as herbalists of yore used to say.

Excessive Menstruation

Normally, only a couple of tablespoonfuls of blood are lost during a menstrual period. However, prolonged vigorous exercise, fibroids, or the hormonal changes of menopause can bring on flooding, which can be rather alarming, and may cause anemia. Excessive bleeding should be checked out by your doctor before you try home remedies—it can be a symptom of endometrial cancer or another serious condition.

Stay off your feet as much as possible the first day of your period—no heavy lifting, and no vigorous exercise. Avoid alcoholic drinks and herbs that stimulate uterine contractions (such as pennyroyal, blue cohosh, and cannabis), and aspirin and other anticoagulants.

If the problem is due to a hormonal imbalance, certain herbal infusions (one teaspoon herb steeped in a cup of boiling water) are said to help: squaw vine and black cohosh for both scanty and excessive bleeding, and licorice root, particularly Chinese licorice, to balance the reproductive hormones. **Warning:** Don't take licorice if you have high blood pressure. A few doctors now prescribe natural progesterone cream or sublingual tablets (placed under the tongue) derived from soybeans or Mexican yams for a variety of "female complaints." Sarsaparilla is also a progesterone source.

Yarrow has been used for centuries to stanch blood flow; Amerindians drank yarrow tea to restore strength after excessive bleeding. Shepherd's purse, a vasoconstrictor, helps control external and internal bleeding (don't take it if you have high blood pressure); amaranth, used for centuries to control hemorrhaging, can also be infused to control bleeding.

Dr. Lucy Smith recommends up to 1,600 IUs of vitamin E to control excessive flow. If breakthrough bleeding disrupts your sleep, take the vitamin at night.

Premenstrual Syndrome

According to the National Women's Health Resource Center, as many as 95 percent of women have some premenstrual discomfort; for 30 to 35 percent of them it is severe. The term "premenstrual syndrome" (PMS) covers a broad range of physical and psychological symptoms. Researchers have not yet pinpointed the cause, but they have discovered that it is more complex than a simple estrogen/progesterone imbalance. Theories that have been advanced but not proven include an excess of prolactin (pituitary hormone) or estrogen; a deficiency of progesterone, vitamin B6, magnesium, or serotonin (a brain chemical); altered glucose metabolism; or altered fluid and electrolyte balance. Dr. James Chuong, Director of Baylor University Medical School's PMS program, has found low levels of beta endorphins (the "feel good" hormones) in women suffering from PMS.

A twenty-to-thirty-minute aerobic workout, on a regular schedule at least four times a week, will increase your production of serotonin and endorphins—relaxation and sleep aids.

Decrease or eliminate your intake of refined sugar, coffee (studies indicate a link with PMS), and nicotine—all stimulants. Alcohol (a depressant) and salt (which increases water retention and subsequent bloating) can also exacerbate your symptoms.

Decrease or eliminate your intake of red meat and poultry; instead, eat lots of fresh fruits and vegetables, whole grains, legumes, nuts, and seeds.

Increase your intake of water, which acts as a diuretic, encouraging your body to eliminate excess fluids.

Take in at least 1,000 milligrams calcium daily, which helps prevent water retention, mood swings, and cramps.

Vitamin C level in the blood drops just before menstruation, so take in extra at this time.

Naturopathic physician Dr. Lucy Smith recommends 100 to 400 milligrams vitamin B6 daily, beginning ten days before the menses to help reduce sugar craving, irritability, and bloating, and 400 to 1,200 IU of vitamin E daily throughout the entire menstrual cycle to relieve breast tenderness and mood swings.

For breast tenderness and other PMS symptoms, the Rhonda Fleming Women's Clinic at UCLA advises evening primrose oil; Take internally, following instructions on the label. Beth Kruse also recommends flax seed and pumpkin seed oils.

Premenstrual Symptom Checklist

Because most women are bound to experience some premenstrual discomfort at one time or another, keeping a premenstrual checklist is a common preliminary to seeking professional help for PMS. The National Women's Health Resource Center suggests charting symptoms, beginning with the first day of your menstrual period and grading them as mild, moderate, or severe. Its list includes abdominal bloating, acne, backache, breast tenderness, constipation, diarrhea, dizziness, fatigue, headache, nausea, swollen hands/feet, anger, anxiety, depression, irritability, nervousness, tension, clumsiness, decreased or increased desire for food or sex, difficulty sleeping or concentrating, forgetfulness, tearfulness, and a tendency to pick fights.

If, after keeping a record for three months, you note that your symptoms consistently increase as the month progresses, particularly between days twenty-one and twenty-eight, you may have PMS. Beth Kruse of Seattle's Aradia Feminist Women's Health Center notes that some women show an increase in symptoms near the tenth day. The key to whether or not you might have PMS, she adds, is an increase in symptoms no earlier than ovulation, and a noticeable drop in symptoms during your period for three out of four cycles.

Dr. Lucy Smith offers these suggestions to PMS sufferers:

- When a patient has PMS symptoms, we often look at the liver, which breaks down nutrients and estrogen so they can be excreted. Herbs and vegetables that improve liver metabolism include beets, carrots, globe artichokes, turmeric, flax seeds, milk thistle seeds, dandelion greens, and dandelion and licorice root teas.

- It is also important to have plenty of omega 6 oils in your diet. Flax seed oil, cod liver oil, and cold-pressed vegetable oils are excellent sources.

- Premenstrual tension and depression may be due to a magnesium imbalance. A co-factor in many enzyme systems, magnesium is depleted by sugar, birth control pills, and stress. Nuts, especially Brazil nuts, sunflower seeds, whole grains, bran, and wheat germ are high in magnesium. If you need supplements, I would recommend 300 to 600 milligrams a day; less if your stools are loose (magnesium is also a laxative). Epsom salts have lots of magnesium. Add a cup to a cup and a half to your bathwater.

- Zinc deficiency can also cause depression and anxiety. You could up your intake by eating nuts, leafy greens, meat, fish, legumes, poultry, seafood, whole grains, egg yolks, brewer's yeast, lima beans, seeds, soybeans, and mushrooms.

- Progesterone builds up in your body during the second half of your menstrual cycle, then stops. Cessation causes your period to begin. Taking in more progesterone can lower your estrogen level, which some researchers believe causes or at least exacerbates PMS. Herbal and vegetable sources of progesterone include wild yam, sarsaparilla, and licorice. The last contains both estrogen and progesterone, but some women find that licorice causes water retention, and it also raises your blood pressure.

- You can also use natural progesterone cream, available in health food stores and some herb suppliers. Apply $1/8$ to $1/4$ teaspoon cream to your breasts if they are fibrous, or to your forearm, stomach, or any part of your body where there is a good blood supply. Sublingual preparations are available.

- Plant estrogens can bring down your estrogen level by blocking the estrogen receptor sites. Alfalfa, don quai, chaste tree, black cohosh, bethroot, and false unicorn root are sources. Foods with estrogenic activity include flaxseed, soybeans, soy flour, and textured vegetable protein. Black cohosh root, blue cohosh root, chaste tree berries, false unicorn root, motherwort, raspberry, and squaw vine tone and strengthen the female reproductive system.

For remedies that treat specific PMS symptoms such as insomnia or nausea, see the appropriate chapter, such as "The Nervous System," "The Digestive and Urinary Systems" (see index).

Pregnancy

At no time of your life is good health and nutrition more essential than when you are carrying and nursing a baby. Vitamin C and A help you resist infections; a high-protein diet gives weight and strength to the developing fetus; folic acid helps protect against some birth defects; and calcium—the amount contained in a quart of milk daily—keeps your bones and teeth strong while your body nourishes the fetal skeletal system and tooth buds.

Coffee and other caffeinated drinks accelerate calcium loss and may cause low birth weight, so use them sparingly—no more than two cups of coffee daily.

How to have a healthy pregnancy
Advice from nurse-midwife Ann Darlington:

- No part of your body will be unaffected by pregnancy. Don't think of the symptoms of pregnancy as aberrations but as part of your greater womanhood. If you anticipate that your body will go through changes, you may be less symptomatic.

- Extra weight is hard on your body, and there's no direct correlation between your weight gain and the baby's size; a link between quality of diet and birth weight is more likely. Eat a diet that is low in sugar and fat and high in dairy products, fruits, and vegetables. An example of a healthy weight gain pattern would be three to five pounds the first trimester, then $1/2$ pound to one pound a week thereafter. If nausea and vomiting are a problem in the first trimester, don't worry about weight gain during that period.

- Some research points to folic acid deficiency as a possible cause of head and spinal cord defects. Folic acid is a component of the B complex that helps prevent birth defects. If your diet doesn't supply it, eat a lot of dark leafy greens. Wheat germ and brewer's yeast are also excellent sources.

- Iron can be hard to digest, and it can cause constipation. If you start out your pregnancy healthy, you may not need iron supplements. However, during pregnancy your blood volume increases by 50 percent. If your hemoglobin level is too low, you run the risk of postpartum bleeding and loss of strength. It's hard to increase iron intake without taking supplements. Every day, especially after twenty weeks, when your blood volume begins to increase markedly, look back on what you have eaten. Iron-rich foods include blackstrap molasses, kelp, broccoli, dark leafy greens, parsley, prunes, raisins, and whole grains. If you didn't get enough iron, take some. Usually 40 to 60 milligrams of "elemental" (absorbable) iron is sufficient for women who are not anemic.

In addition to the nutrients, Dr. Lucy Smith recommends vitamin B12, zinc, digestive enzymes, and high-protein meals.

Herbal and Folk Remedies

AT LEAST a daily cup of raspberry leaf tea strengthens and tones your uterine muscles.

Morning Sickness

Nausea, usually the sign of a healthy pregnancy, can last as long as sixteen to eighteen weeks.

Coping with nausea
Nurse-midwife Ann Darlington has these suggestions:

- Morning sickness is a misnomer; only about 25 percent of the nausea in pregnancy occurs early in the day; another 25 percent occurs in the evening, and the rest is diffuse throughout the twenty-four-hour day. In any event, by the second trimester you are less likely to be troubled by this symptom.

- If you do feel sick in the morning, keep a cracker by your bedside and eat it before you get out of bed in the morning.

- Gingerroot, which studies show is effective at relieving nausea, is helpful to some women. Others find it makes them feel worse.

- Early on, nausea may be related to anxiety. Relax, heed your body, and be sure to get enough exercise and rest.

- Eat small, frequent meals rather than three big ones, so your stomach is never empty or distended, and your blood sugar level is constant.

- Avoid caffeine, alcohol, chocolate, and spicy or acidic foods.

- Take in liquids and solids at separate times.

- If cooking odors or other strong smells bother you, wear nose plugs.

- Prenatal vitamins, specially formulated for pregnant women, can make you queasy. You can safely eliminate them during the first six to eight weeks of pregnancy, even up to twenty weeks if you are really having problems digesting. Vitamins taken with meals are less nauseating. Remember, these are supplements and are generally redundant if your diet is adequate.

- Vitamin B6 helps prevent nausea. Take 200 milligrams over a twenty-four-hour period: 50 to 100 milligrams with food four to six hours or more before you usually experience nausea (e.g., at bedtime if you feel nauseous in the morning), 25 to 50 milligrams at other times. Don't expect to feel better immediately—it takes forty-eight hours for B6 to take effect, and it may initially increase nausea if taken on an empty stomach. **Warning:** An overdose could be toxic to your nervous system, and it will not alleviate nausea. Two hundred milligrams a day is not considered toxic. If you prefer to get your vitamins from food, eat wheat germ, spinach, sunflower seeds, walnuts, brewer's yeast, whole grains, meat, fish, eggs, poultry, carrots, and peas.

- Vitamin E, essential for maintaining a healthy reproductive system, is also helpful in banishing nausea.

- Cloth and Velcro Seabands, available at some pharmacies, health food stores, and nautical shops, enclose your wrist at the acupressure points for nausea and provide relief to some pregnant women.

Herbal and Folk Remedies

BLACK TEA with milk, raspberry leaf tea with cream, or a tea of peppermint or peach tree leaves are universal folk remedies.

IN INDIA and the Middle East, pregnant women scratch and sniff the skin of a fresh lemon to relieve nausea. Keep a lemon in your purse for instant relief.

Sex and Orgasm

The strength of your sex drive is an expression of your vitality; this vital energy is an indication of how well you take care of yourself.

Exercise improves circulation to your sex organs along with the rest of your body, releases endorphins (the "feel good" hormones), tones and strengthens the muscles you use for a sexual encounter, and enhances your attractiveness. Yoga is a particularly apt form of exercise because it improves circulation, glandular function, and suppleness. Tantric Yoga is specifically related to sexual intercourse.

A diet high in protein, loaded with fresh fruits, vegetables, and whole grains, and rich in super-foods (legume and alfalfa sprouts, brewer's yeast, wheat germ, yogurt, and liver) nourishes the glands involved in making love and reproduction, and keeps you energetic and attractive. The B vitamins in the above foods, and vitamin E, found in grains, seeds, and cold-pressed vegetable oils, are most important to your sexuality. Vitamin E is beneficial to your reproductive system, including uterine and vaginal tissue. Food that is raw, unprocessed, and organically grown is highest in vitamins and minerals.

Stress, fatigue, tobacco, and alcohol sap your energy and interfere with your fullest enjoyment of most activities, including sex.

Aphrodisiacs

For centuries, a variety of substances, ranging from the gruesome (bits of moldering corpse) to the sublime (pearls dissolved in wine) have been ingested as a prelude to intercourse. The list of aphrodisiac foods is long and includes stimulants such as chocolate, as well as high-mineral, high-protein dainties such as raw oysters.

Since ancient times, ginseng has been prized in Asia as the supreme aphrodisiac. Although it would not be strictly classified as such, because it does not stimulate the genitals directly, ginseng is a tonic for the glandular system. For women, Dr. Lucy Smith recommends Siberian ginseng because it has yin, or feminine tonifying action.

Damiana, saw palmetto, yohimbé, and kavakava are said to be true aphrodisiacs. Kavakava should be infused and refrigerated for twenty-four hours before drinking. Most spices are also considered aphrodisiac because they provoke tingling in the urogenital tract. A cup of ginger tea is a reputed aphrodisiac. Herbal aphrodisiacs are taken like other herbs: 1 teaspoon dry or two teaspoons fresh herbs to one cup water. Boil roots, seeds and bark and steep leaves for at least ten minutes in boiling water.

A cream containing celandine poppy, cow parsnip, savory, peppermint, and plantain, applied directly to the genitals, is said to help.

Aromatic oils such as peppermint, anise, clove, and wintergreen, diluted with vegetable oil (about ¼ teaspoon aromatic oil to ½ cup vegetable oil) and applied directly to the genitals, produces a warm, tingling sensation that can be very erotic. They are also slightly anesthetic and may help a male partner maintain an erection. These aromatic oils can cause a rash in people who are sensitive to them. To be sure the oils won't irritate your genital area, you should patch-test an area of your mucous membrane first.

Sexercises

Any exercise that improves your flexibility and circulation can in-hance your sexual responsiveness. Exercises that focus on the pelvic area are specifically designed to improve intercourse and orgasm.

Bioenergetics, a Western form of body conditioning that has been compared with Yoga, was developed by Arthur Lowen to restructure, relax, and energize the body for achieving full orgasm. Deep-breathing techniques increase blood oxygen level and energize the body. Lowen used a "breath-ing stool," consisting of a two-foot-tall kitchen stepladder with a tightly rolled blanket strapped to it for padding. Leaning back against the stool encourages deep breathing, as does arching your back while standing or sitting in a low-backed chair.

Kegel exercises were developed by Arnold Kegel, a professor of gy-necology at the University of Southern California who was trying to help pa-tients regain bladder control. Some patients discovered that they were also having orgasms for the first time. The reason is that the muscles responsible for bladder control, the pubococcygeous, or P.C., also contract during or-gasm. Strengthening these muscles increases sexual response for both part-ners. The exercise is simple: while lying, sitting, or standing, take a deep breath and contract your perineal and vaginal muscles as if you were trying to stop the flow of urine. Try to "lift" the contraction of your external mus-cles up into your vagina. Hold for as long as possible, then repeat several times a day for sexual as well as urinary health. You can also do the exer-cise while sitting on the toilet by stopping and starting the flow of urine. This exercise helps tone your vaginal muscles after childbirth and helps all women prevent the loss of bladder control that often begins in middle age.

Physical therapist Elizabeth Noble, author of *Essential Exercises for the Childbearing Years,* describes this sexercise:

> In your coital connection of choice, legs spread and relaxed, grip the penis as tightly as you can with your vagina and hold for a cou-ple of seconds. Relax and repeat the contractions, then rest and try again. With practice, orgasm may occur without direct clitoral stim-ulation.

Postpartum Sex

Timing and problems with postpartum sex
Nurse-midwife Ann Darlington offers this advice:

• After childbirth, your cervix must repair itself, and the placenta site must be given time to heal. The process of sloughing off damaged cells and blood is indicated by the color of your postpartum flow—when the flow no longer has any red, pink or brown tones, the wound has probably completed its healing.

• If you have had stitches, wait at least three weeks after delivery to make love, so that the sutures can be broken down, sloughed off, or absorbed by your body.

• If you feel no pain when you gently palpate your perineum and the inside of your vagina, you are probably ready to accept penetration. Knowing that it won't hurt helps you feel more relaxed and your partner less worried about hurting you.

• Pregnancy is possible even before your menstrual periods return. Since ovulation usually proceeds menses by two weeks, by the time you have your period you are at least one ovulation behind. Therefore don't count on your period as the sole indication of the return of your fertility cycle.

• Periods after your first postpartum one may be regular or irregular in their cycling—both patterns are normal. Your periods may take a while to rebalance.

• It is common to have low hormone symptoms postpartum. These may include vaginal dryness, decreased libido, and depression. These tend to improve gradually and are also linked with other stressors in postpartum life, the most common being sleep deprivation. If you think your imbalances are abnormal, or they are worrisome to you, contact your health care provider.

Vaginitis

A change in the color, consistency, or odor of normal vaginal secretions, itching, burning, or other discomfort may be an indication that you have some form of vaginitis. Hormonal changes, pregnancy, birth control pills, stress, sitting around in a wet bathing suit, or wearing underpants that don't "breathe" can predispose you to an inflammation or infection of the vaginal tissues. Douching, which can change the pH of the vaginal environment and wash away friendly flora, can also create a favorable environment for vaginitis, as can antibiotics, which can destroy beneficial organisms but not yeast. Toilet habits or sexual techniques that transfer *E. coli* bacteria from your rectum to your vagina and unprotected sexual contact are common ways of transmission. Some infections can be serious, so check with your health care provider before trying home remedies.

While you are healing, keep the area clean and dry. To avoid irritation, wear loose cotton underpants, or none at all, and skirts or loose pants. Avoid activities that might irritate the infection such as intercourse, cycling, or inserting tampons.

To relieve external itching, add one cup vinegar or baking soda to your bathwater or apply calendula cream topically to your labia.

Your partner should be treated as well. If you have trichomoniasis or another sexually transmitted infection, this is a must.

To prevent recurrence, follow the treatment for at least two to three days after your symptoms have disappeared.

Unless you and your partner are both healthy and monogamous, when you resume sexual activity practice safer sex by using latex barriers such as condoms.

Bacterial vaginosis (also known as garderella, hemophilus, or nonspecific vaginitis)—

As the name indicates, this is a bacterial infection. It results from a shift in the ecology of your vaginal flora and is sometimes associated with pelvic inflammatory disease. Symptoms, if there are any, include a thin or watery white or grayish discharge and a fishy odor that becomes stronger when mixed with blood or semen. This infection is most likely to show up at the end of your menstrual period. It is typically treated with antibiotics, but the infection may run its course without treatment.

Advice from Beth Kruse, C.N.M., A.R.N.P., and
Aradia Feminist Women's Health Center in Seattle:

Insert a size 00 or 000 gelatin capsule filled with boric acid deep into your vagina twice a day for seven to fourteen days.

Peel a garlic clove, being careful not to nick it, then wrap it in gauze and insert it in your vagina once a day. Leave it in for twelve hours. Do this for three days; on the fourth, douche with vinegar (see below). Repeat the sequence for eight to sixteen days.

About Douching . . .

The healthy vaginal tract cleanses itself; douching is necessary only when you have a familiar infection. Too much water pressure can force unhealthy organisms up into your normally sterile uterus, so insert the nozzle only about an inch and raise the bag only slightly. A reusable latex bag does the job very nicely. **Warning:** Do not douche if you are pregnant. Aradia's Beth Kruse also warns that there is some evidence that douching may sometimes be responsible for more serious pelvic infections.

Douche Recipes for Treating Bacterial Vaginosis

- Vinegar douche: two tablespoonfuls white distilled vinegar to one quart distilled water.

- Yogurt douche: mix two or three tablespoonfuls live lactobacillus culture into one quart distilled water. Keep the yogurt douche refrigerated, warming to room temperature only the portion you will use immediately.

- Salt douche: one tablespoon kosher salt, dissolved in a little hot water, to one quart distilled water.

- Alternate the salt and vinegar douches every other day for a week or two. On the last day, replace the salt or vinegar douches with a yogurt douche. Repeat the sequence if necessary.

- Douche with one part hydrogen peroxide (similar in chemical composition to the cleansing mechanism of a healthy vagina) to eight parts water once or twice a day for a week.

- Use one teaspoon to two tablespoonfuls povidone iodine per quart distilled water once or twice a day for seven to fourteen days. Some women are allergic to iodine, so before you douche with it, test a spot on the back of your hand to see if irritation develops.

- If you prefer not to douche, sit in hip-deep bathwater to which douching ingredients have been added, and take the solution into your vagina by scooting back and forth in the tub. You could also soak a tampon in the solution and leave it in overnight.

Trichomoniasis

Caused by a single-celled protozoan that attacks the urogenital tract, "trich" is usually transmitted sexually, but you can pick it up from using a wet towel or bathing suit recently worn by an infected person. Symptoms, when they are present, include a discharge that is frothy, slightly greenish or yellowish, and has an unpleasant odor. Itching and irritation may be mild to severe. The antibiotic metronidazole (Flagyl) is commonly prescribed, but an early or mild infection may respond to one of the herbal treatments below. If not, do see a doctor.

Douche or take a sitz bath every day for a week using one tablespoon each goldenseal and myrrh or kosher salt to a quart distilled water.

Steep one ounce of the herb St. John's wort in a quart of boiling water for twenty minutes. Strain, add water to make one full quart, and douche with it once or twice daily for a week or two.

Using the preceding recipe, substitute three tablespoons chickweed for the St. John's wort, steep ten minutes, and proceed as directed.

Yeast Infections

Caused by a fungus (most commonly *Candida albicans,* which multiplies and overwhelms the beneficial vaginal flora), these infections are most likely to occur before your period. Symptoms, when they are present, include a thick, caked, or clotted discharge with an odor of freshly baked bread and the consistency of cottage cheese. Itching is the most common symptom. Contributing factors include menstruation, pregnancy, birth control pills, contraceptives, hormonal changes, change in vaginal pH, antibiotics, tampons, tight clothing, and douching. Yeast infections are sometimes associated with depressed immunity and often found in women with diabetes or AIDS.

Dairy products; sugar, and foods that contain it, such as fruit juices; fermented foods (beer, wine, and cheese); and starches, which are changed to sugars by digestion, can aggravate or even help create a yeast infection. However, eating plain acidophilus yogurt every day has been shown to prevent yeast infections.

Letha Hadai, a New York City herbologist and acupuncturist, warns against tea, which is fermented and can encourage the growth of yeast. Herb teas, which are not fermented, are acceptable. Hadai goes on to say, "A tea substitute that will kill yeast is Australian tea tree oil. It can be taken a drop at a time in a cup of water." Tea tree oil is sold in health food stores and herbal outlets.

University of Munich studies have shown that drinking echinacea tea regularly (about $1/2$ teaspoonful steeped for ten minutes in a cup of boiling water) prevents yeast infections. Dr. Lucy Smith advises that echinacea is more effective if you take it only every other week.

Nurse-midwife Ann Darlington notes that postpartum yeast infections are common. Irritation doesn't always indicate an infection; it could be chafing from sanitary napkins. For mild yeast infections before delivery, she recommends acidophilus capsules; after delivery, acidophilus yogurt or boric acid capsules can be effective. However, Darlington adds, if you have not adequately healed and/or are still bleeding, check with your health care provider before putting anything into your vagina.

Douching with a 50 percent solution of fresh aloa vera gel and distilled water, or a teaspoonful of pao d'arco soaked overnight in a quart of cold water reportedly kills yeast cells. If you douche with pao d'arco, drink a hot infusion of the herb (one teaspoon herb to one cup boiling water) at the same time.

Insert acidophilus or goldenseal in size 00 or 000 gelatin capsules deep into your vagina once or twice a day for a week or two.

Try the boric acid treatment described in the BACTERIAL VAGINOSIS section (page 39). Some women find it helpful to insert two of the same size capsules of lactobacillus acidophilus at the same time. Lactinex, found in health food stores and food co-ops, is recommended because of its purity.

To three cups boiling water add four teaspoons calendula (marigold) or St. John's wort, steep ten minutes, strain, add distilled water to make one quart, and use as a douche once or twice a day for a week or two.

To the same amount of water add one tablespoon goldenseal and myrrh or two to three tablespoons bayberry bark; simmer twenty minutes; strain; cool; add water to make a quart; use once or twice daily for a week.

The Digestive and Urinary Systems:

From Constipation to Urinary Problems

t he complex network of glands, nerves, hormones, and enzymes that serves as your body's food processor is intimately connected with all of your other organ systems, which it cleanses and nourishes.

As you chew your food, salivary enzymes convert starches to sugars; in your stomach, digestive enzymes and gastric juices reduce the rest to liquid. Sugar and alcohol pass directly into the bloodstream through your stomach walls. In your small intestine, pancreatic and intestinal enzymes and liver bile complete the digestive process. Digested food is absorbed into your circulatory system through the intestinal walls. Your kidneys filter waste material from your bloodstream and transform it to urine, which is carried to your bladder. The urine passes from your body through the urethra. Indigestible solid waste passes to your large intestine, then is excreted through your anus.

Any part of this intricate metamorphosis can be sabotaged by stress. Rich, fatty foods, which remain in the stomach longest, slow the process down. Exercise speeds it along.

Dr. Beth Schorr-Lesnick, an Attending in Gastroenterology at Beth Israel Medical Center in New York City and Assistant Professor of Medicine at Albert Einstein College of Medicine in the Bronx warns that while many common gastrointestinal disorders respond to self-treatment, consulting your health practitioner is urgent if you are over forty years of age and have a family history of cancer, particularly gastrointestinal or reproductive malignancies; if you drink and/or smoke heavily; if you experience difficulty swallowing, or have unexplained anemia or weight loss.

Constipation

Infrequent bowel movements and/or dry, hard stools are often the result of unhealthy lifestyle and eating habits. They can also be caused by hormonal changes during adolescence, pregnancy, menopause, or aging. Stress and lack of exercise are often contributing factors.

The importance of a daily bowel movement is a matter of some dispute. Some medical experts, including Dr. Schorr-Lesnick, consider one or two evacuations a day to one every five days to be normal if the abdomen is not distended or uncomfortable. Other health professionals, most often naturopaths, herbalists, and other alternative medicine practitioners, believe that if the body is not continually cleansed of wastes through the circulatory, urinary, and digestive systems, it may become toxic.

Relieving constipation

Gastroenterologist Dr. Beth Schorr-Lesnick offers this advice:

- Certain medications such as opiates and other painkillers, tranquilizers, and other psychotherapeutic drugs can slow digestion, including bowel action. Check with your health care professional if you think this may be a problem.

- Regular use of laxatives, particularly stimulants, may damage neurons in your bowel or cause smooth-muscle atrophy. After a while your intestines become dependent on these laxatives and cannot function without them.

- Exercise speeds all processes of digestion, including elimination, so make walking or some sort of workout part of your daily routine.

- The usual dietary undesirables—red meat, chocolate, fried foods, processed foods, breads and pastries made with white flour—can be binding, as can cheese and other dairy products, iron and calcium supplements, and a low-fiber diet.

- Dietary fiber provides bulk. Be sure to eat lots of raw fresh fruits and vegetables, whole grains, and bran. Asparagus, beans, lentils, and most dried fruits are high in fiber. Sunflower seeds, apple juice, and prunes, which stimulate the intestinal walls to contract and secrete fluids, are especially good for you.

- Bran in any form should always be accompanied by liberal amounts of water. Drink at least two quarts of water or other fluid daily.

- Pain from anal fissures or hemorrhoids can inhibit a bowel movement. Stool softeners, plenty of fluids, and a high-fiber diet can ease the pressure.

- If dietary strategies for constipation don't work for you, try milk of magnesia, magnesium citrate, mineral oil, Fleet enemas, or glycerin suppositories.

- Call a doctor if the constipation persists for more than a week or two; if there is bleeding, distention, or pain; or if laxatives produce vomiting rather than evacuation—you may have a bowel obstruction or other serious medical condition.

Nurse-midwife Ann Darlington notes that magnesium deficiency can sometimes cause constipation. Be sure you get enough of this mineral in the form of nuts, dried fruit, whole grains, or rice.

Daily abdominal massage also helps elimination. In a light, brisk, counterclockwise motion, describe tiny circles around first your navel, then your lower abdomen, centered just above the pubic bone, and finally your upper abdomen just under your breasts. Spend about one minute massaging each area, then gently knead your abdomen.

Herbal and Folk Remedies

MANY ALTERNATIVE medical practitioners believe that certain foods and herbs increase the flow of bile; improve liver, stomach, and gallbladder function; and relieve constipation. Globe artichokes, rhubarb, chicory, fiddlehead ferns, olive oil, and all parts of the dandelion serve this function. Helpful herbs include peppermint, garlic, milk thistle, marigold, lavender, linden, yarrow, yellow dock, and gentian.

PSYLLIUM, THE principal ingredient in some commercial laxatives, and flax seeds provide bulk and soften the stools; licorice and hibiscus teas and fresh cucumbers or watermelon are gently laxative.

FOR SEVERE constipation, herbalists sometimes recommend a teaspoonful of the herb senna steeped in boiling water for ten minutes. Senna should be taken with an equal amount of fennel, mint, cinnamon, or clove to help expel gas and avoid griping. Dr. Schorr-Lesnick cautions that senna is a stimulant laxative and, for reasons previously given, should be used sparingly. **Warning:** Do not take any laxative if you experience abdominal pain or tenderness or if you are pregnant or nursing.

THE JUICE of one lemon in a cup of hot water taken before breakfast is all some people need to establish regularity. An apple a day is also excellent health insurance. The fruit is rich not only in fiber but in pectin, which restores the function of the large bowel. Raspberries are also laxative. Blueberries have the interesting quality of both loosening and tightening the bowels: raw blueberries relieve constipation; the dried berries help arrest diarrhea.

CARIBBEAN REMEDIES include the herb cerasee (available in health food stores), aloe vera, and a mixture of olive oil and lemon juice.

RUSSIANS TAKE two tablespoons of honey in a cup of boiling water once a day.

A POPULAR African remedy for constipation is ripe papaya taken with meals. In stubborn cases, papaya seeds are ground to a powder; then a teaspoon or two is mixed with coffee or tea and taken before breakfast for two days. Another papaya remedy is two or three teaspoonfuls of the liquid that is released when a cut is made in the skin of a ripe papaya. This is mixed with two teaspoonfuls of honey and taken orally as often as needed.

Diabetes

Diabetes is a serious chronic disease involving abnormal or insufficient secretion of insulin and high levels of sugar in the blood. Early symptoms include inordinate thirst and frequent urination, weight loss, and general malaise. Insulin is given to control the symptoms.

In the early stages of diabetes, dietary strategies may be sufficient. Non-insulin-dependent diabetes, which occurs most often in overweight adults, may be managed with diet and exercise. Daily exercise helps keep your weight down and improves all digestive processes, including glandular activity. The most important dietary strategy is to avoid sugar and starches, which are changed to sugar in the digestive process, and to refrain from overeating. Eat six small meals a day rather than three large ones to help regulate your blood sugar. **Do not undertake self-care, however, until you have consulted a doctor.**

Infections can lead to grave complications when you have diabetes, so it is important to avoid them by practicing good hygiene and dealing promptly with cuts and abrasions.

Herbal and Folk Remedies

INCORPORATE GLOBE and Jerusalem artichokes into your meals. Although these delicious vegetables are not botanically related, both contain inulin, a starch that is not converted to sugar in the digestive process.

RODALE PRESS, in a booklet, *The Good Fats,* reports that purslane, a fleshy, mucilaginous plant that grows all over the world, has been shown to reinforce the body's own insulin supply.

The American Botanical Council and Herb Research Foundation Report:

- The herb fenugreek is said to have an anti-diabetic effect.

- Legumes, garlic, raw onions, and licorice can slow adult diabetes.

- USDA studies show that insulin activity is tripled by ingesting cinnamon, cloves, turmeric, or bay leaf.

CLINICAL STUDIES indicate that sage tea may lower blood sugar levels in diabetics. Some herbalists recommend tea made with blueberry leaves, Chinese licorice, yarrow, or nettles to reduce blood sugar levels. Ginseng tea is also recommended for diabetes. **Herbs for such a serious condition, especially ones as powerful as these, should be taken only under the supervision of a health care professional trained in their use.**

A CARIBBEAN remedy is a cup of ginger tea (one teaspoon powdered or two or three slices fresh to a cup of water) taken upon arising in the morning and at bedtime.

Diarrhea

Diarrhea can accompany common viruses and flu or result from food poisoning or food allergies. The frequent, watery bowel movements serve to eliminate disease microorganisms, toxins, or irritants. Unless it is severe, lasts more than a few days, or is accompanied by fever or blood in the stool, a bout of diarrhea probably should be allowed to run its course. Persistent or frequent episodes of diarrhea should be checked by a doctor—it could be a symptom of a serious condition.

Controlling diarrhea
Advice from gastroenterologist Dr. Beth Schorr-Lesnick:

- When you have diarrhea, limit your diet to rice and bananas. Both are binding, and bananas are rich in potassium, a mineral often eliminated along with fluids when you are suffering from diarrhea.

- If you have cramps, limit your food to clear gelatin and drink only clear fluids such as broth or soup so your bowels can rest. Avoid fruit juices, which are laxative.

- Prolonged diarrhea can be dehydrating. Tissue salts are lost along with fluids, and the resulting disturbance of the electrolyte balance can be debilitating or life-threatening. To replace these vital nutrients, add a pinch of salt and a pinch of bicarbonate of soda to a liter of water. Drink several cups a day for the next few days to restore electrolyte balance. Gatorade and similar sports drinks also supply missing tissue salts.

- Take two tablespoons Pepto-Bismol or Kaopectate or four tablespoons Imodium. Imodium and Pepto-Bismol are more effective if they are taken together. If your tongue or stools turn black, don't be alarmed—it's a harmless side effect of taking Pepto-Bismol.

- Lactose intolerance can cause chronic diarrhea. Many adults, especially those of Asian or African descent, lack the enzyme lactase, which digests the lactose in milk and other dairy products. Yogurt with active cultures supplies the missing enzyme and is usually tolerated by people who are lactose-intolerant.

- See a doctor if (1) your symptoms persist for more than a few days; (2) there is blood in the stool; (3) you have a high fever. If diarrhea is accompanied by weight loss, the problem could be food poisoning or malabsorption (nutrients not passing through the intestinal wall). **Consult your health care professional.**

Since the turn of the century, scientists have known that the lactic-acid-producing bacteria found in yogurt and other cultured milks can treat intestinal problems. Recent research has confirmed that *Bifodbacteri bifidum,* found in breast milk and some brands of yogurt, and *Streptococcus thermophilus,* also found in yogurt as well as in other cultured milks, prevent spread of infant diarrhea by reducing the excretion of the rotavirus that caused the diarrhea. As a preventative, many people eat yogurt with live acidophilus cultures every day. The beneficial flora not only help maintain colon health, but also comprise the bulk of the feces.

A daily quart of yogurt with live cultures can replace beneficial flora that are wiped out along with disease bacteria when you take antibiotics. In this way you may avert diarrhea caused by the demise of friendly flora.

Herbal and Folk Remedies

CHARCOAL ABSORBS toxins, including those that cause diarrhea. If you don't have charcoal in your medicine cabinet, burned toast is a source.

RICE, the water rice has been cooked in, sweetened with sugar, or cream of rice cereal can arrest a mild attack.

THE PECTIN in apples helps restore normal bowel function if you have diarrhea.

THE HERB goldenseal, which is sold in health food stores, contains berberine, which is antimicrobial. Take ½ teaspoon goldenseal in a cup of boiling water.

ASTRINGENT HERBS dry up the watery secretions that cause diarrhea. Tannin, both astringent and healing, can be found in Chinese tea (green tea, especially Gunpowder and Dragon Well, is an ancient Chinese remedy). Other sources of tannin include witch hazel, tormentil, plantain, white oak bark, and the leaves of strawberries, blueberries, raspberries, and blackberries. Dried blueberries and blackberry brandy are also good.

IN THE HIMALAYAS, nutmeg is used to treat diarrhea. The spice is also used in Aruyvedic medicine for the same purpose because it is astringent and sedative, drying up intestinal secretions and suppressing the muscular contractions that cause bowel movements. Nigerians use black pepper to treat intestinal disorders.

FATHER JOE HEALEY, a Maryknoll priest who has spent nearly 30 years studying folk culture while a missionary in Tanzania, notes that dried, ground papaya seeds are the most popular remedy for amoebic dysentery, a severe form of diarrhea. He has personally experienced papaya's efficacy and recommends a teaspoonful of ground or fifteen whole seeds three times a day for ten days. Garlic, he adds, is another popular Tanzanian remedy for intestinal infections. "A man I know takes garlic every day."

IN INDIA, Father Joe recovered from a bout of constipation after taking juice from the bel tree. The priest who recommended the cure claimed that bel was the greatest medicine he had used in all his life, for the bel also dried up diarrhea. "In fact," the priest told Father Joe with a mischievous grin, "bel juice has the power of sacred scripture: it can bind or loosen."

Traveler's diarrhea
Some tips from gastroenterologist Dr. Beth Schorr-Lesnick:

- Avoid tap water, ice made from tap water, and foods washed in it. Boiled water is usually safe to drink.

- When considering whether a food is safe to eat, use this rule of thumb: peel it, boil it, cook it, or forget it. Cucumbers you peel yourself are probably safe, but not salads made with raw fresh vegetables, or fruits.

- Tea made with boiling water may be okay; bottled drinks are better; carbonated beverages are the best.

- Researchers have discovered that if you begin taking Pepto-Bismol as directed two to four times a day when you arrive at your destination, you are 50 percent less likely to suffer from diarrhea. Be aware that Pepto-Bismol may turn your tongue or stools black.

- If you do get diarrhea while traveling, take Pepto-Bismol together with Imodium as directed. If you have high fever and bloody diarrhea, discontinue the Imodium and see a doctor.

- Casual use of antibiotics is not recommended because of possible side effects. However, if you are traveling on business and have no time to be sick, you could bring antibiotics with you and take a three-day course at the first symptoms of diarrhea or dysentery. Ask your physician for advice on this.

- Replace fluids and tissue salts with the salt and soda mixture described on page 49, with Gatorade or a similar sports drink, or, if you are traveling in a Third World country, with rehydration packets supplied by the United Nations.

Dyspepsia

Indigestion, which just about everybody gets at one time or another, is usually the result of eating too much fatty, fried, or acidic food. Sometimes it is caused by hormonal changes commonly experienced during pregnancy and menopause, or by stress, aging, or even serious illness. Consult your health care provider if the bouts are frequent or prolonged.

Some indigestion can be triggered by a food allergy or intolerance. Identifying and eliminating the culprit may be all that's necessary.

Taking digestive enzyme tablets before meals or eating foods containing digestive enzymes as part of the meal is another strategy. Pineapples, papayas, and papaws contain digestive enzymes; so does papaya leaf tea.

Herbal and Folk Remedies

MOST CULINARY herbs and spices are digestives, so use them liberally in cooking. For example, allspice and ginger are popular in the Caribbean for indigestion and stomachache. The Middle Eastern culinary herb fenugreek is often prescribed by herbalists for dyspepsia, poor appetite, and general debility.

SINCE ANTIQUITY, people have taken bitters before a meal to increase the flow of saliva and gastric juices that aid digestion. Infusions of gentian, wormwood, and Oregon grape were often used. The English herbalist Samuel Culpepper's recipe calls for two teaspoons sliced gentian root, two teaspoons dried orange peel, and four tablespoons dried lemon peel infused for an hour in a pint of boiling water; take four tablespoonsful three times a day. Your local supermarket probably sells bitters; add a dollop to your aperitif.

MANY AFTER-DINNER liqueurs and sweets contain stomach-settling herbs such as anise, fennel, calamus, angelica, caraway, gentian, ginger, or peppermint.

IN THE CARIBBEAN, three or four leaves of the indigenous herb yerbabuena is steeped in a cup and a half of water. The dose is a cup a day.

IN CHINA, oolong tea has been sipped for centuries to relieve indigestion.

Gas and Flatulence

Advice from gastroenterologist Dr. Beth Schorr-Lesnick:

Many people are overly concerned about the frequency with which they pass gas—an average of fourteen times a day is within the normal range.

Stomach gas and flatulence can result from swallowing air while chewing gum, eating too fast or with ill-fitting dentures, or talking while eating. Breaking these habits may cut down on your gas.

Eat slowly, under relaxed conditions, if possible, and chew your food thoroughly. If you have recently switched to a high-fiber diet with lots of fresh fruits and vegetables, legumes, and bran, you may experience gas and flatulence for two or three weeks, until your digestive system adapts. While your body is adapting, try cooking these foods until they are quite soft so they are more digestible and less gaseous. Embarking on a raw-food diet can have similar results. Introduce raw foods gradually and chew them well.

A food diary is a very useful tool in solving dietary problems. To keep such a diary, simply write down everything you eat, including amounts; whether the food is cooked or raw; when you ate the foods; any reaction you may have had and how long it lasted.

After a couple of weeks, try eliminating the items that cause discomfort, one by one, to see if your symptoms improve. Certain foods and drinks are notorious gas producers: carbonated beverages, lentils, legumes, beans, and members of the cabbage family. If you don't want to eliminate these foods, it may help to take Beano, an anti-flatulence product sold in supermarkets, before you eat them. Adding a pinch of baking soda to beans and lentils before they are cooked is a traditional strategy.

Although their reputation as flatulent foods is less well known, bagels, breads, pasta, and other wheat products, corn, oats, and potatoes may also be culprits. Carbohydrates are likely to ferment in your gastrointestinal tract, creating gas in your stools.

Many adults, especially those of Asian or African descent, cannot manufacture lactase, the enzyme that digests lactose. In consequence, such people cannot digest milk, resulting in gas, cramping, bloating, and diarrhea. Some dairies now produce milk that supplies the missing enzyme. Yogurt, which contains lactase, and some hard cheeses "predigested" by bacteria or enzymes can usually be tolerated.

You may have gas if food remains in your stomach too long. Certain medications and foods can slow emptying: painkillers, tranquilizers, and antidepressants; chocolate, caffeine, and fats. Eliminating as many of these foods and drugs as feasible may correct your digestion.

Gas and flatulence can also be a symptom of a medical disorder such as a weak lower gastroesophageal sphincter muscle or incomplete emptying of the stomach, perhaps due to an ulcer or cancer. It is important to consult a medical professional if you are over forty years of age, have a family history of cancer, experience loss of appetite or weight, or have blood in the stool or black stools.

Gaviscon, Maalox, Mylanta, and activated charcoal may be effective over-the-counter remedies for heartburn and gas.

Exercise improves your abdominal muscle tone, allowing you to control the release of gas.

Herbal and Folk Remedies

MOST AROMATIC herbs expel gas from the intestines by stimulating intestinal movement. Fennel or anise seeds, peppermint leaves, and gingerroot are four of the best. They can be taken as teas or after-dinner cordials. Traditionally, candied ginger has been served after a meal to promote digestion and help expel gas. You might also try cinnamon and other spices, mustard, pepper, dillseed, wintergreen, chamomile, caraway, or garlic.

A YOGA gas-expelling technique is to lie on your stomach with one leg tucked under you so your knee is against your chest. Hold this position for a few moments, then repeat, raising the other leg. Do this until you have expelled the gas.

IN THE Caribbean, camphor is soaked in water and used as a warm compress to reduce gas pain. In Jamaica where it grows, an entire cerasee plant, including the seeds, is boiled for twenty to thirty minutes in a pint of water, then the water is sipped by the teaspoonful.

Hangover

The aftereffects of overindulgence in alcohol are all too familiar: a headache that just won't quit, often accompanied by nausea and sometimes diarrhea. Smokers, who tend to consume more tobacco when they drink, especially at social gatherings, are likely to feel worse the morning after than their non-smoking fellow revelers. Since the effects of overindulgence tend to be short-lived, and the discomfort is unlikely to require medical attention, most hangover remedies are anecdotal and fall into the realm of folk medicine.

An old-fashioned preventative is to coat your stomach by drinking a glass of milk before you embark on an evening of drinking. Later, as you imbibe, remember that alcohol passes into your bloodstream more slowly when it is accompanied by food. Eating protein while drinking is particularly good for delaying alcohol absorption.

Some people avert hangovers by taking a couple of aspirin and a lot of fluid at bedtime. If you are one of those unfortunates who gets terrible hangovers from drinking red wine but persist in the habit anyway, take two Advil before indulging and two more at bedtime.

Nausea and vomiting, which eliminate alcohol toxins, should be allowed to run their course unless they become prolonged or severe.

Certain vitamins are depleted by drinking bouts: A, E, and the B complex. If nausea or diarrhea is not a problem, a hearty breakfast is all some people need to set them on their feet. Many people drink tomato juice or a bloody Mary the morning after to replenish vitamin B6, which can control nausea. Some drink Coca-Cola or breakfast on raw oysters with Worcestershire sauce, a universal mainstay.

Jamaicans mix soda water with bitters, used for centuries to restore digestion, or sip ginger tea with the peel of an entire orange.

A traditional morning-after cure is "the hair of the dog that bit you." Alcohol does serve as a mild muscle relaxer and tranquilizer, but habitual use can lead to a vicious cycle of resorting to either the dog or the hair.

Heartburn

Regurgitation of gastric juice into your esophagus can result in the burning sensation in your chest and breastbone area known as heartburn. Esophageal spasm and gallbladder inflammation also produce heartburn symptoms, so it is wise to check them out with your health care professional if you have frequent episodes or a prolonged one.

Relieving heartburn
Gastroenterologist Dr. Beth Schorr-Lesnick has this advice:

- Certain substances trigger overproduction of stomach acids, directly irritate the gut lining, weaken the gastroesophageal sphincter, or delay stomach emptying. These things include tobacco, chocolate, peppermint, coffee and other beverages containing caffeine, calcium channel blockers, Valium, citrus fruits, tomatoes, and fried or fatty foods.

- Other possible causes include a lax gastroesophageal sphincter, poor gastric emptying, or reflux action.

- Contrary to what you might expect, neither a glass of milk nor baking soda (sodium bicarbonate) is the answer. The calcium in milk triggers the release of gastric acids, and the combination of acid and baking soda (you may have used it as a leavening agent) could cause your stomach to burst.

- Clothing that is tight, especially around the waist and stomach, can add to your discomfort by forcing stomach acids into your esophagus. Obesity can produce a similar effect.

- Small, frequent meals require less gastric acids for digestion and are emptied more quickly than three big ones, thus helping you avoid heartburn.

- To allow the digestive process to get under way, don't recline after a meal or eat less than two hours before you sleep or exercise. When nighttime heartburn is a problem, elevate the head of your bed or use a wedge to elevate your upper body.

- If none of these strategies help, consult your doctor.

Lying on your right side increases the backflow of stomach acid into the esophagus, so keep to the left.

According to a *New York Times* report, Dr. Walter L. Peterson of the University of Texas Southwestern Medical Center notes that wine and beer stimulate excess stomach acids; hard liquor does not, and may be a safer choice if you must drink alcohol.

Teresa Carr, writing in *American Health* magazine, reports that a large glass of cold water will wash the acid back into your stomach and help dilute it when it is there.

Sucking on hard candy increases your saliva production and neutralizes acids.

Ginger, a folk remedy popular in areas as diverse as China and the Caribbean, is an excellent stomach settler, digestive, and acid neutralizer. Boil the entire root in about a pint of water and drink the broth, chew a piece of the root, nibble a piece of crystalized ginger, or take a capsule or so of the powder.

Hemorrhoids

Also called piles, these are actually varicose veins outside or just inside the anus. Because of hormonal factors early in pregnancy, carrying additional weight, and straining at delivery, many women suffer from hemorrhoids during pregnancy and childbirth. Stress, overindulgence in alcohol, and constipation can aggravate the condition, which is uncomfortable at best and at the worst painful and sometimes bloody.

Avoiding and relieving hemorrhoids
Advice from gastroenterologist Dr. Beth Schorr-Lesnick:

• Truckdrivers and other people who sit a lot, dancers, weightlifters, overweight people, and others who lift or carry extra pounds often suffer from hemorrhoids. Usually the swollen tissue is not painful unless a blood clot has formed in the vein. Bleeding is not necessarily cause for alarm, but it can also be a sign of rectal or colon cancer, so be sure to check it out with your health care professional, especially if you are over forty or have a family history of cancer.

• Protracted coughing and sneezing can cause hemorrhoids, so treat these conditions promptly with the appropriate medications if they are caused by allergies or colds.

• Avoid constipation and straining to pass stools. Fats and refined foods slow digestion and elimination, which can foster or aggravate hemorrhoids. Take in lots of fluid and a high-fiber diet that includes fresh fruits and vegetables, dried fruit, bran, and legumes. Stool softeners such as psyllium and flaxseed can be helpful. (See also CONSTIPATION, pages 44–47.)

- Don't read while sitting on the toilet —it encourages you to linger in a position that may foster hemorrhoids.

- Bathe your hemorrhoids thoroughly to avoid itching. Witch hazel pads help keep the area clean and shrink tissue. To ease irritation, sit in a lukewarm shallow bath three or four times a day with water up to your hips. Adding a cup of Epsom salts helps heal the inflammation. If you use a basin that fits in your toilet seat

for your sitz bath, add a tablespoonful of Epsom salts. (Nurse-midwife Ann Darlington suggests hot sitz baths with Epsom salts to stimulate blood flow to the area and reduce swelling. Follow the hot bath with a cold one to shrink the tissue.)

- Hemorrhoid suppositories or anesthetic creams and sprays may also help relieve irritation.

- If the problem doesn't clear up in a couple of weeks, see a doctor.

Certified nurse-midwife Ann Darlington advises:

- Try not to bear down when evacuating. If you have a problem with constipation, take an enema if necessary.

- Avoid peppers and spices, which irritate sensitive anal tissue.

- Exterior hemorrhoids are the most painful because the sphincter muscle constricts the engorged blood vessel. Apply a little olive oil and, lying or leaning over with your hips elevated, try to push them back inside.

Short of surgery, which sometimes must be repeated a few years later, some experts believe the best remedy for exterior hemorrhoids is to stretch the sphincter muscle. You can do this with a special implement designed for the purpose. Natural foods and alternative health care magazines advertise it.

Herbal and Folk Remedies

ADVERTISING HYPE to the contrary, nonprescription over-the-counter preparations don't shrink hemorrhoidal tissue—they only lubricate it. You need an astringent such as witch hazel to reduce the swelling. Dip a clean cloth in a mixture of one part witch hazel and one part ice water. Elevate your hips while lying or leaning over and apply the compress for fifteen minutes after every bowel movement, and every couple of hours the first day, then two or three times a day until you obtain relief.

STEEP TWO teaspoons each of black tea and comfrey in a cup of boiling water. Refrigerate the mixture after it cools, and alternate a tea compress with the witch hazel compresses. The tannin in the tea and the comfrey forms a protective film over the wounds, and the allantoin in the comfrey heals by speeding the formation of new skin cells.

SOME PEOPLE obtain relief by drinking tea made from tormentil root, which is sold in health food and herbal outlets.

Intestinal Parasites

Although children are more likely than adults to get worms, these parasites can infect an entire family. Children get them by playing in the dirt, then transferring the eggs to their mouths. Once a child is infected, the eggs can be passed on to other family members by sharing bed linen or towels. Some worms, such as the hookworm or tapeworm, cause serious symptoms such as weight loss or anemia. Others, such as the pinworm, the most common, mainly cause itching and scratching, but the irritated skin can become infected.

Strict hygiene is essential to prevent spread of infection. Launder clothes in hot water and germicide and make sure all family members wash their hands thoroughly and frequently, especially before eating.

Herbal and Folk Remedies

MOST DRUGSTORE preparations for killing worms are toxic to a degree. For centuries, herbalists have used plants to accomplish this purpose. They are said to work better if you take them in the morning, after fasting.

WORMWOOD, AS the name implies, was a major vermifuge. The oil, which is released in alcohol, was once the basis for absinthe, notorious for its destructive effect on the nervous system. Infused wormwood is quite effective against intestinal worms, and not harmful to humans because the toxic oil is not released in water. Herbalist David Hoffman, in *The Holistic Herbal,* recommends steeping a teaspoon or two of the dried leaves in a cup of water for ten or fifteen minutes. Sip a cup three times a day.

RAW GARLIC has proved effective against intestinal parasites since the time of the ancient Egyptians. Eat as much of it as you can.

PUMPKINSEEDS WERE an official worm medicine until after the turn of the century. The dose is a half cup, to be taken in the morning after a night's fast. Since the seeds paralyze the worms but don't kill them, follow the seeds with a strong laxative or enema to expel them from the intestines.

IN AFRICA, several fresh, washed cabbage leaves and a little water are brought to a boil. The juice is squeezed from the leaves and two or three teaspoons are taken every day. Papaya is used for another African remedy. Grind the seeds to a powder, mix with coffee or tea, and take before breakfast for a couple of days. You could also score the skin of a ripe papaya and collect the juice that is released. Mix two or three teaspoons of this liquid with two teaspoons honey. Repeat the dose until the worms are expelled in the stools.

Irritable Bowel Syndrome

If you have alternating bouts of constipation and diarrhea, with considerable gas and bloating, chances are you may be suffering from irritable bowel syndrome. The origins of irritable bowel syndrome have yet to be pinpointed, but stress and tension are thought to exacerbate or precipitate attacks. For treating the constipation and diarrhea, see the appropriate sections, pages 44–47 and 48–51 respectively.

Coping with irritable bowel syndrome
Dr. Beth Schorr-Lesnick has these suggestions:

- Some people are hypersensitive and may have an abnormal perception of abdominal distention. True irritable bowel syndrome does involve bloating and discomfort and frequently colon spasms as well, but some hypersensitive people may perceive as abdominal distention what is actually only minor discomfort. If you have chronic intestinal upsets and fluctuations with no accompanying fever to indicate infection, you should consult your doctor.

- Some people, especially those of African or Asian descent, do not manufacture the enzyme that digests milk lactose. Lactose intolerance can result in the symptoms described above. Eliminating dairy products from your diet, replacing milk with yogurt, or taking oral lactase tablets may solve the problem. Try one of these strategies for a couple of weeks and see if it helps.

- Gluten, a protein found in wheat, and to some extent in rye, barley, and oats, can cause similar problems in people who cannot digest it. Eliminate these grains from your diet and stick with corn and rice for a couple of weeks to see how your gastrointestinal system reacts.

- Psyllium seeds, the main ingredient in Metamucil and similar preparations, are high in fiber. They can stabilize the bowel condition by providing bulk and softening the stool.

- Irritable bowel can also result from a fluid imbalance in the intestines. When your intestinal walls secrete too much fluid, you get diarrhea; too little, and you are constipated. Equalactin, nonprescription tablets sold in pharmacies, equalizes the water content in the large intestine. Taking in plenty of fluid is also helpful.

Herbal and Folk Remedies

∙∙

TORMENTIL, A wild European plant, is often prescribed by herbalists for alternating constipation and diarrhea. Steep a teaspoonful in a cup of boiling water and take by teaspoonfuls throughout the day.

EAT APPLES—they help restore the function of the large bowel.

Liver Function

This hardworking gland performs more than five hundred functions, including detoxifying and purifying the blood and regulating its chemistry; storing fat, glucose, vitamins, and minerals; processing estrogen; and producing bile. The largest gland in your body, the liver plays a key role in digestion and can be damaged by an overload of alcohol and rich, greasy foods. Because your liver performs so many functions, it can bring about a wide range of health problems when it malfunctions, from skin problems and a general feeling of malaise to jaundice and hepatitis.

**Gastroenterologist Dr. Beth Schorr-Lesnick,
a specialist in liver malfunction, offers this advice:**

- A high-fat diet, obesity, starvation, diabetes, or an excess of fat-soluble vitamins A, D, E, and K can result in excess fat in your liver. Avoid cooking oils such as palm or coconut, and stay with the polyunsaturates such as safflower oil or monosaturates such as olive or canola. If you are diabetic, you must avoid sugar—among other problems, you may suffer from fatty liver.

- Too much animal protein in your diet can stimulate your liver to overproduce ammonia, which may result in confused thinking and other mental problems. Control your liver's ammonia production by getting your protein from vegetables and dairy products.

- Overloading your liver with salt may result in water retention. Avoid salty condiments and cold cuts. Lemon juice is the best salt substitute.

Herbal and Folk Remedies

IN CHINA, the herb astragalus is used to protect the liver against damage by toxic drugs.

MILK THISTLE has been clinically tested and shown to be successful at treating amanita mushroom poisoning, hepatitis, and cirrhosis.

DAILY PRACTICE of yoga helps regulate the glandular system.

JAMAICANS TAKE a daily tablespoonful of olive oil as a liver cleanser.

IN SPRINGTIME, people the world over who live in areas where dandelions grow feast on the greens. Gathered young, gently steamed, and dressed with butter or olive oil, garlic, and a dash of lemon or vinegar, the spinach-like potherb is a folk remedy for liver disorders and just about anything else that might ail you. It provides an epicurean treat and a wealth of vitamins, minerals, digestive bitters, and important enzymes.

Mouth and Tooth Problems

Indigestion? Gas? The problem may originate in your mouth, where dental misalignments, missing teeth, or ill-fitting dentures can interfere with chewing. The digestive process begins as you chew your food. By taking the time to reduce your food to the smallest particles, you spare the rest of your digestive system extra work and reduce gas and flatulence.

Bleeding Gums

Bleeding gums are most often caused by either gingivitis, a surface infection of the gums common during pregnancy, or pyorrhea, a chronic gum infection that can result in bone loss under the gums.

Coping with gum disease
*Reola Moss, Dental Hygienist at Long Island College Hospital Dental Clinic,
in Brooklyn, New York, has these suggestions:*

- For the infection to heal, it is important to keep your teeth and the surrounding tissue scrupulously clean. Floss daily, and clean between your teeth with a tiny brush designed for that purpose.

- Brush your teeth with a soft-bristle toothbrush and a paste made by mixing baking soda and peroxide.

- Using your finger, massage your gums daily to stimulate circulation.

Herbal and Folk Remedies

SPRINKLE SOME powdered myrrh (sold in herb and health food stores) on top of your toothpaste before you brush your teeth. The herb is a natural resin, antiseptic and astringent, good for bleeding gums and combating the infection that causes them. Some dentists recommend tincture of myrrh to patients with periodontal problems.

ELIZABETHAN HERBALISTS recommended garlic to "fasten loose teeth"—loosened, no doubt, by gum disease. Rubbing a cut garlic clove over your gums won't improve your breath, but it can dispatch the microbes responsible for gingivitis and pyorrhea.

Canker Sores

These small, hard swellings on the tongue or inside the mouth were formerly thought to be a reaction to stress or certain allergens such as citrus fruits, chocolate, nuts, or aged cheese. Although cankers remain somewhat of a medicinal mystery, says otolaryngologist Melissa Pashcow, it is likely that they are an infection.

Cankers eventually heal themselves, Dr. Pashcow says, but they can be quite uncomfortable while they last. She recommends washing your mouth with equal parts water and peroxide two or three times a day until the canker goes away. Any mouth sore that does not heal should be evaluated by your doctor.

Herbal and Folk Remedies

···

BAKING SODA, milk of magnesia, and other antacids neutralize bacterial and viral secretions and make the site less painful.

AN OLD country remedy is to steep the herb goldthread in a half eggshell and apply to the canker.

GOLDENSEAL, MYRRH, and oak bark are traditional remedies for mouth sores. The first two are antiseptic as well as astringent. Moisten the dried herb with a little water and apply directly to the canker.

Toothache

An impacted wisdom tooth or a gum abscess can be a source of pain, but usually the cause is a cavity that results from tooth decay. Thorough cleaning and a calcium-rich, sugar-poor diet are sensible preventative measures.

Herbal and Folk Remedies

···

DROP CLOVE oil directly into the cavity. Oil of peppermint is also anesthetic, but clove seems to be more effective.

A SCOTTISH remedy is to roll a few drops of whiskey in pepper to form a smooth ball, then insert the pepper ball in your aching tooth.

JOURNALIST CATHERINE Clifford reports that Ronald Melzack and Dr. Kenneth C. Bentley, a Montreal, Canada, researcher and oral surgeon, advise rubbing the web of skin tissue between your thumb and forefinger for about five minutes with an ice cube wrapped in a gauze pad. The tissue is an acupressure point for stimulating endorphins, and the intense cold, says Melzack, may activate a mechanism in the brain that temporarily inhibits pain messages from the tooth.

THE ROOTS of California poppies contain alkaloids that are chemically similar to opium. Amerindians inserted a piece of the root into the cavity of an aching tooth to relieve pain.

Tooth Decay

Small amounts of a natural chemical that helps prevent cavities are present in plums, raspberries, strawberries, endive, cauliflower, and eggplant. The Seneca Indians used to brush their teeth with mashed strawberries; eggplant charcoal is used in some dentifrices sold in natural food stores.

Nausea and Vomiting

Nausea, and subsequent vomiting, is often linked to the nervous system—from the queasy feeling that may accompany nervous tension to vomiting provoked by noxious odors, disturbing sights, or severe pain. Flu, food poisoning, or overindulgence in alcohol or food—especially fats and sugars—can trigger vomiting as the body attempts to throw off toxins. Many women experience nausea during the first trimester of pregnancy. Loss of equilibrium due to motion sickness or a middle-ear infection can make you nauseous; so can grave illnesses such as diabetes and certain cancers.

Unless vomiting is severe or prolonged, it is best to let it run its course to get rid of toxins, bacteria, or indigestible foods.

Avoid acidic foods, advises gastroenterologist Dr. Beth Schorr-Lesnick. Orange juice is worse than whole oranges, she says; tomato products and foods with strong aromas, such as fish, are notoriously bad. She recommends small portions of salty items such as saltine crackers and white and yellow foods such as plain pasta, cheese, and bread and crackers, which may be easier to keep down.

Coping with nausea
Dr. Karen Lawson, a Minneapolis internist, has this advice:

- Find out why you are sick. Try to remember what you ate. Nausea can be an early symptom of food poisoning or appendicitis. If your temperature is over 101 degrees or the nausea is accompanied by abdominal pain, see a doctor immediately.

- Avoid further insults to your stomach by taking only clear, sweetened liquids such as 7UP or ginger ale for the first twelve hours. (Water and other fluids that contain no salt or sugar won't stay down.) Gatorade and similar sports drinks are helpful in replacing salts and sugar lost in vomiting.

- Acupressure relieves nausea. Make a fist with your left hand. Note the two tendons that pop up on the inside of your wrist, running from the base of your palm to your elbow. Bend your wrist and press your right thumb three fingers' width below the crease in your wrist, on the outside of the tendons. Press down firmly for a minute, then move your thumb up to your wrist and press for another minute. Mild queasiness may be relieved immediately. More intense nausea may require twenty minutes of repeated pressing.

- Seabands, which are cloth and Velcro bracelets sold in pharmacies and health food stores, press on acupressure points for nausea. They do work for morning sickness.

- Chamomile tea is also good for stomach upsets, unless you are allergic to ragweed—a close botanical relative.

Herbal and Folk Remedies

GINGER HAS a centuries-old reputation for relieving nausea and other stomach disorders. The Herb Research Council reports that it is used in a London hospital for postsurgery nausea. Apparently, ginger interrupts communication between your stomach and the nausea center in your brain. Chew on the root or boil the root in a pint of water for about thirty minutes, strain and sip as needed.

A TEASPOON of goldenseal steeped in a pint of boiling water and sipped by the teaspoonful brings some people relief.

OTHER ANTI-NAUSEA herbs that have been used in folk medicine include peppermint, spearmint, anise, cumin, caraway, clove, ginseng, chamomile, raspberry leaf, and lavender.

IN INDIA and the Middle East, people scratch the peel of a fresh lemon and sniff the aroma to relieve nausea.

A SCOTTISH recipe for beef tea to restore strength after nausea: Cube one pound of lean steak, season with salt and pepper, put in a stone crock, cover, and place in a pan of water halfway up the jar. Bring the water to a boil so the meat will steam for three hours, strain, and sip the broth.

Motion Sickness

The dizziness and nausea associated with traveling in a moving vehicle or vessel, whether through water, in the air, or on land, is actually a matter of equilibrium. According to the American Academy of Otolaryngology, an association of ear, nose, and throat physicians, our sense of spatial orientation is based on sensory input from our inner ears, eyes, skin pressure receptors, and muscle and joint sensory receptors. You can experience motion sickness when your central nervous system receives conflicting messages—for example, your muscle, joint, and skin receptors feel turbulence, but your eyes do not detect this motion because you are inside a boat or plane.

Preventing and/or relieving motion sickness:
The American Academy of Otolaryngology has these suggestions:

- Always ride where your eyes will see the same motion that your body and inner ears feel. For example, sit in the front seat of a car and watch the scenery, or the deck of a ship and gaze at the horizon. When airborne, sit in a window seat over the wing.

- Don't face backward or read while traveling.

- Avoid strong odors and spicy or greasy foods immediately before and during travel.

In laboratory studies, ginger proved as effective as Dramamine at relieving motion sickness. Chewing on the fresh root or taking a capsule or two of dried, powdered ginger root should do the trick.

Dr. Karen Lawson, a Minneapolis internist, recommends a couple of folk remedies—Coke syrup and 7UP. Most people don't have Coke syrup on hand, she says, but uncarbonated Coke, or even root beer, is acceptable. Pour the soft drink into a large bowl and let it sit for a few hours until it goes flat. Take small amounts slowly—up to two tablespoons every ten minutes. It helps to sip through a straw because it slows you down.

Ulcers

Peptic and duodenal ulcers are an inflammation of the mucous membranes lining the stomach and duodenum. The symptoms are a burning sensation and pain; sometimes the ulcer breaks through the stomach or intestinal wall and becomes a perforating ulcer. Ulcers are associated with stress and were thought to be caused by excess stomach acid. Current medical theory points to infection, with acid as a permissive factor.

Gastroenterologist Dr. Beth Schorr-Lesnick notes that there are no specific foods to avoid, but spicy, tomato-based, and citrus foods are common irritants. She suggests keeping a food diary (see page 53) to record your reaction to individual foods—an important strategy in dealing with gastrointestinal symptoms.

Although milk and cream used to be recommended for ulcer diets, they may actually be the culprits in creating ulcer pain. Calcium stimulates the production of stomach acids, Dr. Schorr-Lesnick says.

Herbal and Folk Remedies

DR. GARNETT Cheney of Stanford University's School of Medicine recommends a daily quart of raw cabbage juice, which can be made in a juicer or blender. Cabbage contains gefarnate, a substance used in anti-ulcer drugs to strengthen the stomach lining and replace cells. It takes about three weeks to see results.

DRIED, UNRIPE plantains—the banana-like fruit popular in Hispanic cuisine—prevented and cured ulcers in rats in a British study.

A RUSSIAN folk remedy is to take a daily tablespoon of honey dissolved in hot water.

CHAMOMILE, USED for centuries in folk medicine, in laboratory studies has been shown to inhibit ulcers in rats. Chamomile is anti-inflammatory and antibiotic, healing to wounds and lesions. Its antispasmodic and sedative ingredients counteract stress. Dr. Rudolph Weiss, author of *Herbal Medicine*, recommends three cups of tea a day (two teaspoons dried herb to a cup of boiling water), to be taken on an empty stomach before breakfast, at midafternoon and bedtime. This must be taken over a period of time, until the ulcer is completely healed. Although most people can take chamomile freely over long periods of time, those who are sensitive to ragweed, a botanical relative, should proceed cautiously until assured there is no allergic reaction.

Urinary Problems

Your kidneys, the approximate color and shape of a kidney bean, are vitally important to your internal health. They filter waste products from your blood, regulate the water content and salt balance of your body, and maintain the acid/alkaline balance of your blood. Drink plenty of water—it helps flush your urinary system of impurities and bacteria.

Kidney Stones

In some people, toxins, excess minerals, and certain acids can accumulate in the kidneys and form gravel and stones. To prevent them from forming, drink plenty of fluids, particularly diuretics, to flush out harmful acids, minerals, and toxins.

Herbal and Folk Remedies

CRANBERRY JUICE, nettle leaves, and all parts of the dandelion are said to help prevent the formation of kidney stones and gravel. Columbine root, birch leaf tea and hawthorn berries are believed to be helpful in breaking up the stones.

Urinary Incontinence

Involuntary urine leakage is usually due to a weakening of the muscles of the pelvic floor. Such leakage happens during pregnancy when the enlarged uterus presses against the bladder. Uterine tumors that enlarge or protrude from the uterus can also press against the bladder, with similar results. Some elderly women have problems with incontinence due to bladder irritation often caused by inflammation.

The most effective preventive is strengthening your pelvic muscles through exercise. To learn to contract your vaginal muscles, sit on the toilet with your legs apart and stop and start the flow of urine. After a while you should be able to clench and unclench these muscles like a fist. This exercise should be done fifty times a day for the rest of your life.

Avoid irritants such as coffee, alcohol and spicy foods, which make you feel you want to urinate.

Herbal and Folk Medicine

DR. RUDOLPH Weiss, author of *Herbal Medicine,* recommends a mixture of the herbs saw palmetto, sweet sumac, and hops, mixed with pumpkinseed oil.

Urinary Infections

A frequent need to urinate coupled with small output, pain, or a burning sensation upon urinating are indications of a urinary infection. The usual culprit is bacteria transferred from the colon to the urinary tract by careless toilet habits, or by sexual practices that involve anal contact directly followed by intercourse. Constipation is also sometimes responsible.

Although urinary infections are usually treated with antibiotics, a mild infection or one in its early stages can sometimes be cleared up with folk remedies or herbs. It is essential, however, that you get a professional diagnosis first.

When you have a urinary infection, it is helpful to drink plenty of water to help flush out bacteria, and to avoid irritants such as coffee, alcohol, and spicy food.

Avoiding and coping with urinary infections
Advice from nurse-midwife Ann Darlington

- To prevent infections, empty your bladder after sexual intercourse. The urine moves *E. coli* (an intestinal bacteria that often causes infections) forward and away from your urethra. Urinate before you make love, then take in some liquid so you can urinate again directly afterward.

- Diaphragm use can encourage bladder infections by changing the location of the bladder and acting as a pessary to inhibit complete emptying.

- After you have a bowel movement, wipe from front to back to avoid introducing bacteria from your bowels into your urinary tract.

- If your physician diagnoses your urinary infection as interstitial cystitis, a painful inflammation in the bladder wall, do not drink cranberry juice, which is ordinarily very good for the urinary tract. The juice helps the bacteria adhere to your bladder wall.

Herbal and Folk Remedies

DIURETICS KEEP your kidneys in good working order by encouraging the flow of urine. Black currant juice, rich in vitamin C, has a diuretic effect. Cucumber and watermelon (especially the seeds), watercress, carrots, nettles, dandelion, chicory, chervil, leeks, onions, asparagus, juniper seeds, celery, parsley, goldenrod, and sorrel are also diuretics and helpful to consume when you have a urinary infection.

IN LABORATORY studies, cranberry juice and blueberries have been shown to inhibit the growth of some bacteria, including *E. coli,* a source of urinary and yeast infections. Cranberry juice has a diuretic effect, is a good source of vitamin C, and also contains quininic acid, which inhibits the formation of kidney stones.

ONE OF the best herbal remedies is bearberry leaves, which you can buy in most health food stores. Soak the leaves in cold water (one teaspoon to one cup water) for twelve to fourteen hours to avoid releasing tannin. Varro Tyler, author of *The New Honest Herbal,* advises that the urine needs to be alkaline, so don't take bearberry with acidic foods. Bearberry leaves, which have a high tannin content, tend to darken the urine. To avoid toxicity, take no more than two or three cups a day for no longer than a week or two.

A RUSSIAN remedy is to drink cranberry juice and bearberry tea, relax pain with two warm baths a day, and sleep with a scarf or other wool covering wrapped around your abdomen.

BARLEY WATER is a Scottish recipe for kidney problems. To make it, combine one cup pearl barley, $^1/_2$ teaspoon salt, and two quarts water. Cover the barley with water and bring to a boil, cover, then simmer until the barley is soft, drain, add salt, and drink cold.

Weight Management

The amount of fat you carry and the way it is distributed owes much to heredity but is finally determined by your eating and exercise patterns. Whether you see yourself as too fat, too thin, or just right, a few basic rules apply:

- Eat six small meals rather than three larger ones to maintain a balanced metabolism and blood sugar level.
- Exercise helps you take off inches and keep them off. If you are underweight, outdoor exercise does wonders for your appetite.
- Avoid sweets, soft drinks, and other foods that offer only empty calories with little or no nutritional value.

Overweight

Although an underactive thyroid can be responsible for obesity, usually people add pounds because they combine too much sugar and fat with too little exercise. Crash diets are rarely successful in the long run because they don't change eating patterns.

Much of the spectacular weight loss in the early part of a diet isn't fat; it's water. Salt attracts fluids, so limiting the sodium in your diet will also limit water retention. Diuretics are part of some reducing diets. Oddly enough, the best one is water. Drinking it encourages urination, so you put out more than you take in. Also, the water dilutes sodium.

Exercising early in the day gets your metabolism going, so you burn off calories more efficiently throughout the day. Yoga is particularly good because the different postures stimulate circulation to particular glands, thus regulating your endocrine system.

A diet high in fiber and carbohydrates gives you a sense of fullness and has fewer calories.

Recent studies indicate that a high-protein diet causes weight gain in some people.

Gastroenterologist Dr. Beth Schorr-Lesnick observes that taking off weight depends on the individual. She recommends a high level of activity, eating smaller portions, and eliminating snacks, food with empty calories, and fatty junk foods.

Herbal and Folk Remedies

HERBALIST LETHA Hadadi recommends certain teas that are used in China for weight loss. Cleansing teas such as Bojenmi, Tuocha, jasmine, and na yen ti kuan yin speed up your digestion and aid your body in utilizing foods more efficiently. Bojenmi contains medicinal herbs said to strengthen your stomach and spleen and reduce water retention, which can be a source of bloating and excess weight.

Underweight

While it may be true that you can never be too rich, a few people *are* too thin. Active younger women sometimes have trouble putting on and maintaining weight, especially in summer when we tend to prefer a lighter diet consisting of more low-calorie fruits and vegetables and less starch and protein.

Gaining weight
Gastroenterologist Dr. Beth Schorr-Lesnick offers this advice:

- Fatty foods help you gain weight. In the short run, eating ice cream won't hurt you. You can also supplement your meals with Carnation Instant Breakfast.

- Rich puddings are also fattening.

- Eat lots of high-protein pasta, whole grains and whole-grain breads, and other complex carbohydrates, as well as healthy snacks and desserts.

The Cardiovascular System:

From Anemia to Varicose Veins

We tend to think of cardiovascular disease as a male disorder. For the first four decades of a woman's life this is usually so because estrogen protects most premenopausal women from coronary disease. In spite of the initial hormonal advantage, however, the American Heart Association reports that the number one killer of American women is heart attack.

A history of hypertension and diabetes early in life makes you vulnerable to cardiovascular disease later on. Women who prefer not to take estrogen replacement therapy should be especially careful to control the risk factors.

The health of your cardiovascular system owes much to your genes, which determine the structure of your blood vessels and how you process cholesterol. A healthy lifestyle is also important.

The American Heart Association, along with other medical experts, points to smoking as your greatest risk factor. The nicotine in tobacco accelerates your heart rate and constricts your blood vessels, raising your blood pressure. Inhaled tobacco smoke raises the carbon monoxide level in your blood, thus robbing your heart and other tissues of oxygen. Women smokers who use oral contraceptives are at even greater risk.

A sedentary lifestyle, intense stress, and/or a diet high in saturated fats also put you at risk for cardiovascular disease. Patients in the Dean Ornish Program for Reversing Heart Disease at Beth Israel Medical Center in New York City have reversed their coronary disease and lowered their cholesterol by eating a vegetarian low-fat diet, engaging in aerobic exercise, practicing Yoga, and relying on group support.

All of these factors, which are discussed later in this chapter, are recommended by most alternative and an increasing number of mainstream medical practitioners as the key to a healthy heart and blood vessels.

Anemia

Menstruation and childbearing make women particularly vulnerable to anemia, a red blood cell or hemoglobin deficiency. Individuals who are more prone to anemia are those who are slender, smokers, or aspirin users. Women who wear IUDs or have kidney problems are also vulnerable to anemia. The level of hemoglobin—the part of the red blood cell that contains iron and transports oxygen to your tissues—tends to drop as you get older. The most common causes of anemia are inadequate iron intake, blood loss through excessive menstruation, and increased blood production during pregnancy. Weakness, fatigue, shortness of breath, and pallor, especially of the inner eyelids, are the most apparent symptoms.

Iron-rich foods are your best preventative. Some authorities state that heme iron, present in beef, poultry, and fish, is more easily absorbed than the non-heme iron present in fruits, vegetables, and grains. Liver, lamb kidneys, and eggs are leading sources of heme iron.

If you don't eat meat, fish, or poultry, it is important to include iron-rich plants in your diet. Dried beans, spinach and other leafy greens including dandelions and nettles, dandelion roots, dried apricots and peaches, sunflower seeds, wheat germ, black walnuts, parsley, and blackstrap molasses are excellent sources of iron. Rice polishings, which are the nutrient-rich outer husks of rice, are also rich in iron. Look for this product in health food stores.

Vegetarians are also at risk for pernicious anemia, which can result from a vitamin B12 deficiency. Few plants have this important nutrient, and the ones that do have very little. Many physicians advise vitamin B12 supplements for strict vegetarians.

It has long been known that a substance similar to hemoglobin has been found in the roots of nitrogen-fixing plants such as beans, lentils, clover, and alfalfa. More recently, scientists in Germany, France, and Australia have suggested that all plants may have the genes to produce hemoglobin for transporting oxygen. Therefore, it might be wise to include more legumes and root vegetables in your diet.

Athletes and others who take strenuous exercise can experience iron loss through sweat. To compensate, you might take extra iron when you expect to perspire a great deal.

Coffee, tea, and other caffeine-containing beverages interfere with iron absorption. Avoid them or at least cut down consumption.

Multivitamin and mineral preparations for pregnant women may contain antacids and fillers that interfere with iron absorption. Vitamin E can also interfere with iron absorption. Karen Parker, writing in the journal *Birthing,* suggests taking iron at bedtime, and eight hours from the time you take vitamin E. To reduce constipation and other side effects, Parker recommends chelated iron, available in health food stores.

Herbal and Folk Remedies

THE HERBS angelica, fenugreek, barberry bark, agrimony, centuary, quassia chips, and raspberry leaves are good sources of iron. Native

Americans boiled the entire yarrow plant and drank it as a blood-building tonic.

AN OLD country remedy for iron-poor blood is to insert a small iron nail in an apple overnight, then eat the apple. A similar strategy is to cook foods in cast-iron pots and pans.

BEER MADE with nettles, a wild plant with stinging hairs that is harvested in spring in many parts of the world as a health-giving potherb, is said to be a good blood builder. The following traditional Scottish recipe is from F. Marian McNeill's *Recipes from Scotland,* published in 1946 by Albyn Press: 3 handfuls young nettles, 2 handfuls dandelion, 2 handfuls cleavers, $1/2$ handful wood sage, 1 ounce bruised whole fresh gingerroot, 1 ounce compressed (baker's) yeast, a piece of toast, $1/2$ ounce cream of tartar. Boil the plants in one gallon water for 15 minutes; strain. Add 3 pounds of sugar and ginger; boil and strain again. Cream the yeast and spread on the toast; float on the lukewarm liquid. When fermented, add the cream of tartar, bottle, and cork. Store bottles on their side in a cool, dark place. If you are impatient for results, omit the cream of tartar and allow the liquid to stand near a fire overnight. Skim and bottle, being careful not to disturb the sediment. The beer will be ready in a few days.

Arteriosclerosis

Arteriosclerosis occurs when your blood vessel walls thicken and harden with deposits of calcium, then fat, making it increasingly difficult for blood to circulate. The narrowed blood vessels cause the blood platelets to stick together and cause clots. If the clot blocks a coronary artery, you have a heart attack; if an artery leading to your brain is blocked, you have a stroke.

Hardening of the arteries is a leading cause of death in Western nations. It is often a silent disease, which increases the danger: you may not show symptoms until the disease is far advanced. When symptoms do appear, they are similar to those of high blood pressure, which is often involved: dizziness, drowsiness, ringing in your ears, muscle cramps, and bluish skin. Whether or not you get arteriosclerosis depends largely on the structure of your blood vessels, which may cause blood flow disturbances.

The American Heart Association states that the higher your total blood cholesterol level, the more likely it is that fats and cholesterol will build up on your artery walls. Recent studies have shown that a cholesterol level under 200 is optimum for our society. The liver manufactures about 500 to 1000 milligrams daily of this waxy white material, some of which is necessary to insulate nerve endings and help produce certain hormones. A high cholesterol level can be due to liver malfunction or genetic factors, but most people's high cholesterol level is due to saturated fat intake.

The American Heart Association advises: avoid saturated fats, including fatty red meats, whole milk, hard cheese, butter pastries, and coconut, palm, and palm kernel oils. Contrary to advertising hype, margarine is not the healthy alternative. Hydrogen molecules, whipped into vegetable oil to harden it, make the resulting product more saturated than butter.

Until recently, people were advised to avoid high cholesterol by eating unsaturated fats. However, recent studies indicate that oxidation of unsaturated fats can produce free radicals—cell-destroying molecules, a suspected cause of cancer and other diseases. Monosaturates such as almond, olive, avocado, and canola oils are the better choice: not only are they more resistant to oxidation, but they actually lower blood cholesterol.

Omega 3 oils can significantly lower your cholesterol level. These oils are present in fatty fish such as mackerel and tuna. They are also found in canola, rice bran, walnut, soybean, and wheat germ oils, and in soybeans, purslane, walnuts, and beechnuts.

You don't need to eat unusual foods to keep your cholesterol level down. Any bulky, high-fiber food may positively affects your blood sugar level and the way you absorb cholesterol. Eat lots of fruits, vegetables, and whole grains. Dried beans, peas, and lentils are your richest source of fiber; bran and dried fruits such as prunes and apricots are also excellent sources.

Antioxidants—i.e., foods or supplements containing vitamins C, E, or beta carotene—are thought to help prevent arteriosclerosis. Vitamin C supplements can raise high-density lipoprotein (HDL)—"good" cholesterol. Lipoproteins "carry" cholesterol out of the arteries to the liver, hence from the body. High-density (HDL) cholesterol has more of these carriers. Your HDL, according to the American Heart Association, should be above 35 milligrams per deciliter. Some people find supplements of vitamins B6 and B12 helpful. Many nutrition-oriented health professionals recommend supplements of the entire B vitamin complex to get the full benefits of these vitamins.

Although heavy drinking isn't good for your heart, one or two drinks a day, especially of red wine, can help maintain low cholesterol. Red wine also contains quercetin, an anti-carcinogen. A positive link between alcohol consumption and breast cancer has been established, however. Women who are at risk might want to weigh this against the possible cardiovascular benefits of a drink or two.

If you drink coffee, make it filtered. A Dutch study revealed that coffee made by steeping the grounds in boiling water raised cholesterol, but filtered coffee had no effect.

Smoking tobacco contributes to hardening of the arteries. According to the American Heart Association, your level of high-density lipoprotein ("good") cholesterol rises when you quit smoking.

Keeping your weight down also helps keep your cholesterol level down. Cholesterol levels seem to rise and fall with weight level, possibly as a consequence of blood fat storage. Weight loss and learning to avoid and manage stress can help lower your cholesterol level. (See pages 73–74 in Digestive System chapter and pages 169–171 in Nervous System chapter for details.) Exercise is an effective way to control both your weight and your stress level. Aerobic exercise that speeds up your heart rate and makes you breathe harder and deeper gives your heart a workout and improves circulation. A brisk walk will also do it—aim for one to three miles a day.

Herbal and Folk Remedies

GINGER IS very beneficial to the circulatory system. Among other functions, it lowers cholesterol and inhibits the platelet clumping that leads to clotting and impedes circulation. A Puerto Rican prescription for healthy arteries is to drink a cup of ginger tea in the morning and at bedtime.

GARLIC, A universal folk remedy that dates back at least five thousand years, has in this century been the subject of several laboratory studies. A 1993 New York University investigation showed that a half to a whole clove of raw garlic daily lowers cholesterol by 9 percent. Other studies show that garlic is beneficial to blood lipid levels; it inhibits blood platelets from sticking together, and reduces susceptibility of blood fat to oxidation.

THE HERB Research Foundation reports that rose oil and vitamin A lower the level of blood lipids that carry cholesterol in your blood. Oolong tea, fenugreek, celery extract, and the pectin in grapefruit peel are said to lower cholesterol.

LINDEN, OR lime blossom tea, a popular European bedtime relaxer, helps protect against buildup of fatty deposits on arterial walls.

JAMAICANS BOIL an entire cerasee plant, including seeds, for twenty to thirty minutes and drink the tea every day to clean out cholesterol. Cerasee, which grows wild in Jamaica, is used in both Asian and Caribbean medicine. Look for it in health food and herbal outlets and Korean markets.

HAWTHORN LEAVES, flowers, and berries have been used since the nineteenth century to treat cardiac conditions, including arteriosclerosis. Pharmacognosist Varro Tyler describes it as a mild heart tonic which research has shown dilates blood vessels and lowers blood pressure.

THE FAN-SHAPED leaf of the ginkgo tree, a staple of traditional and folk medicine in China and India for thousands of years, has been the object of recent Harvard and University of Virginia studies. Ginkgo has been shown to improve blood flow in cerebral arteriosclerosis and successfully treat irregular heartbeat.

Cold Hands and Feet

Cold hands and feet are usually inherited, and not cause for concern. If your fingers or toes turn dead white, a sign that the small arteries supplying blood to the fingers and toes are temporarily constricted, or if you experience pain while walking, you could have a vascular disease and should consult a physician. In most cases, cold hands and feet are more a nuisance than a danger.

The quickest way to deal with cold hands and feet is to put on your hat. Since most of your body heat escapes from the top of your head, capping it prevents heat loss. In chilly weather, covering your neck and wrists will keep your major arteries warm so blood circulates freely.

Mittens are better at keeping your hands warm than gloves, but do wear thermal gloves under the mittens. Warm wool socks and thermal inner soles or thermal boots help keep your feet warm.

Vitamins B6, B12, and E help protect your vascular system. To make sure you get enough of these important vitamins, include nuts, seeds, and whole grains, especially wheat germ, in your daily diet.

Omega 3 oils, found in fatty fish such as mackerel and tuna, beans, soybeans, beechnuts, butternuts, walnuts and canola, rice-bran, soybean, walnuts, and wheat-germ oils, also improve circulation by thinning your blood.

Keep your fingers and toes moving. Such Exercise stimulates circulation.

The Scleroderma Society has these tips for people who are particularly sensitive to cold:

- Put rubber caps on your keys, doorknobs, and other cold objects, especially metal ones.
- Use a napkin or fabric holder for cold drinks.
- Warm up your car before driving; use fabric seat covers and a steering wheel cover.
- Put on mittens before you handle cold metal or open the refrigerator.
- Wash vegetables and hand laundry in tepid rather than cold water.

Herbal and Folk Remedies

WARM UP with a cup of ginger tea. Ginger improves circulation by inhibiting the release of prostaglandins, body chemicals that cause the blood platelets to stick together.

CAYENNE PEPPER has a similar effect. Taken internally, cayenne warms you up and stimulates circulation. Sprinkle some in your socks and mittens to warm your hands and feet.

Hypertension

The main causes of high blood pressure are calcium and cholesterol buildup, which narrows the arteries, and fluid retention by the kidneys, which increases the volume of blood, so the heart must beat more forcefully to circulate it. Genetic predisposition is a major factor, but lifestyle habits also contribute. Like arteriosclerosis, which often precedes it, hypertension is a silent disease until it is quite advanced. If your blood pressure is high for an extended period of time, you have an increased risk of stroke, heart and kidney disease. (The normal range varies with age and other factors, but the American Heart Association defines high blood pressure as "readings of 140/90 or greater that stay high over an extended time.") Although most patients have no symptoms, you may experience headache, dizziness, blurred vision or ringing in your ears.

Dr. Dahlia Garza , Attending in Cardiology at Beth Israel Medical Center in New York City, on high blood pressure:

Hypertension may increase your risk for coronary disease, and long exposure to high blood pressure, if left untreated, can injure your heart. Young women should address high blood pressure before it becomes a problem. The effects of high blood pressure are insidious; over time it can lead to coronary artery disease, kidney failure, or stroke. It's very important to control this disease and take your medication if you need it.

Since there are basically no symptoms of high blood pressure, it's important, as you age, to have your blood pressure monitored as part of your regular medical care. Both smoking and taking birth control pills can increase your risk for blood clots and stroke.

Although salt is not ordinarily harmful to a healthy person with no kidney problems, it does cause fluid retention, which increases blood pressure.

Losing weight and exercising could be a first step toward lowering your blood pressure. Vigorous exercise does raise your blood pressure temporarily. This can be dangerous if your hypertension is uncontrolled, but if you are careful and on medication, you should be able to safely engage in exercise.

Stress doesn't cause high blood pressure, but it does exacerbate it. Choose an exercise that relaxes you—walking and swimming are great, yoga even better.

Risk factors for hypertension
Advice from the American Heart Association:

Pregnancy increases your potential for high blood pressure (because, as midwife Ann Darlington points out, your blood volume increases significantly).

Heredity and race are potential risk factors. If members of your family have had heart disease, you are more likely to develop it. Black Americans have a greater risk of heart disease than white Americans—in large part because they have higher average blood pressure levels.

Menopause is another risk factor. Nearly half the women over 55 have high blood pressure.

You are at high risk if you are overweight or take certain oral contraceptives.

Meditation, visualization, and other relaxation techniques can help you manage stress. For details, see pages 169–171 in Chapter Seven, "The Nervous System." Massage helps you relax and gently stimulates circulation. In addition, researchers have found that after a thirty-minute massage, subjects had consistently lower levels of the stress-related hormones cortisol and norepinephrine.

Herbal sedatives work on the central nervous system, helping your entire body relax. Some used most often are valerian root and skullcap, passion flower, hops, hawthorn, lavender, blue vervain, birch, blind nettle, celery, lettuce, peach, and linden leaves. Linden is also believed to help regulate circulation.

Replace salt with herbal seasoning or lemon juice. Most prepared foods contain sodium, so read the labels first to discover which ones are salt-reduced or salt-free. You should be able to find low-sodium and sodium-free foods in the health foods or special dietary section of your supermarket.

Keep your weight down. Studies show that losing weight is even more vital to lowering blood pressure than is lowering salt consumption.

Eliminate saturated fats, which build up on your artery walls and narrow your blood vessels, raising your blood pressure and making your heart work harder.

Omega 3 oils can significantly lower blood pressure. You'll find them in fatty fish such as mackerel, salmon, and tuna. Other omega 3 sources include soy and other dried beans, walnuts, purslane, canola, rice bran, and wheat oils.

Lowering cholesterol with a high-fiber diet that includes fruits, vegetables, and whole grains helps prevent fatty buildup in the arteries.

For more information on controlling cholesterol, see pages 78–81 in the ARTERIOSCLEROSIS section.

Folk and Herbal Remedies

DIURETICS ARE usually prescribed for hypertension patients. If your blood pressure is only slightly raised, you may be able to lower it with gentle diuretics, which include dandelion greens and "coffee" made from the root, parsley, strawberry leaves, cleavers, sarsaparilla root, raw cucumber, lemon juice, hops, whole celery, cranberry juice, watercress, and plain water. In the Caribbean, one buchu leaf is steeped in $^1/_2$ cup boiling water.

CELERY EXTRACT is thought to lower blood pressure. Dr. John Lust, author of *The Herb Book,* claims that celery seeds are sedative and the entire plant diuretic. Celery does have a high sodium content, however. The herbs yarrow, guelder rose, wood betony, elder flower, and hibiscus are also said to help lower blood pressure.

THE FLOWERS and berries of hawthorn, a botanical relative of the apple, have been used since the nineteenth century to regulate circulation. Hawthorn is said to dilate the blood vessels, regulate heart action, and lower blood pressure.

GARLIC HAS been shown to significantly lower blood pressure. Jamaicans take a daily tablespoonful of chopped raw garlic clove with an equal amount of olive oil. Other Jamaican remedies are a wineglassful of whole cucumber juice or alfalfa tea, and tea made from cerasee, an indigenous plant used in both Asia and North America for a variety of ailments.

Jamaicans also boil the entire cerasee plant, seeds and all, for twenty to thirty minutes, and drink the tea daily to bring down blood pressure.

IN BELIZE, onions are boiled in vinegar and the resulting broth drunk.

RUSSIANS DRINK a half glass of beet juice daily.

Low Blood Pressure

Cardiologist Dr. Dahlia Garza on low blood pressure:

A lot of people are overly concerned about low blood pressure, but you shouldn't be as long as your blood pressure profuses (supplies blood to) your organs completely. A low blood pressure reading is not necessarily a pathology; it may require no treatment. In fact, if you have low blood pressure when you are young, chances are you won't suffer from high blood pressure when you get older. Young, slender women tend to have lower blood pressure.

Hypotension is important only if it affects vital organs. There will be overt symptoms: you'll feel cold and clammy and woozy. If you have low blood pressure that's a problem, you should be treated by a doctor immediately, as it is a life-threatening illness.

Dangerously low blood pressure (which should be treated immediately) is one way your body may respond to an emergency, but not to a chronic condition. In an extreme allergic reaction, for example, histamines cause the blood vessels to open up and widen. Abnormal widening of the blood vessels can lead to extreme low blood pressure and cardiovascular collapse.

Malnutrition or exhaustion can lower your blood pressure, but, again, these are rather extreme circumstances. The remedy is fairly obvious: be sure you get enough rest and sleep, and eat sensible meals that include lots of fresh produce; whole grains; and nuts, seeds, and other high-protein foods.

Vigorous aerobic exercise raises your blood pressure temporarily. It also improves circulation, gives you energy, gets rid of tension, and improves your appetite and digestion.

Folk and Herbal Remedies

BITTERS SUCH as gentian, wormwood, Oregon grape, and goldenseal can stimulate your appetite and improve digestion. If your blood pressure is low because you lack important nutrients, these help.

IF STRESS and nervous exhaustion are the problem, try an herbal sedative such as skullcap, valerian, passionflower, hops, peach leaf, or lavender.

HAWTHORN FLOWERS and berries act as a heart tonic, normalize circulation, correct palpitations, and act as a gentle sedative.

LICORICE RAISES the blood pressure, at least temporarily. You might try eating licorice candy, chewing on licorice root, or drinking tea made from the boiled root.

Lymphatic System

Thin, yellow lymph fluid flows in tiny channels between your cells and through the lymph glands located in your neck, underarms, groin, and breasts. The two main functions of your lymph system are fighting disease and cleansing your lymph fluids, then returning them to the bloodstream— a process that was formerly known as "purifying the blood."

Alternative health practitioners believe that cleansing your tissues of toxic material is essential to a healthy lymph system. They suggest you avoid red meat and greasy, fatty, sugary, processed, or adulterated foods.

Try a cleansing diet for a week or more, limiting your consumption to fresh, raw fruits and fresh juices. Later, add fresh greens, then other vegetables, and finally nuts, fish, and poultry if desired.

Folk and Herbal Remedies

A SOAK in Epsom salts is an old-fashioned strategy for drawing out wastes and toxins. Add a cup to a hot bath, then immerse yourself up to your neck until the water is cool. The bathwater may be tinged yellow—a sign that cleansing has taken place.

CERTAIN HERBS are reputed to stimulate elimination of tissue waste. These include cleavers, goldenseal, marigold, sarsaparilla, devil's-claw, burdock, figwort, blue flag, yellow dock, and nettles.

ECHINACEA GIVES powerful support to your immune system, helping you avoid infection. Take about a half teaspoon a day in capsule or decoction form. Dr. Lucy Smith, a naturopathic physician, advises taking the herb every other week for best results. In this way, your immune system does not become dependent on this powerful herb.

Palpitations

Some heartbeat irregularities, such as an occasional skipped heartbeat, can be normal. The fluttering, throbbing, and poundings of the heart known as palpitations are common reactions to emotional or physical stress. You get them when your heart is overactive. Anxiety or nervousness may be the cause. Excess secretions from the adrenal or thyroid glands, menopause, or low blood sugar can also result in palpitations. They are seldom cause for alarm, but they could be a sign of anemia or low blood pressure. If you have a history of cardiovascular disease, or if the palpitations are accompanied by a fall in blood pressure and light headedness, you may have a problem, so check with your doctor.

If your heart flutters after drinking coffee or smoking a cigarette, limit your intake of caffeine and nicotine. Sugar may also cause palpitations. If your sweet tooth proves irresistible, at least balance your sugar consumption with some protein. Better yet, replace sugar with complex carbohydrates.

Avoid rich foods and large meals. Fruit, vegetables, whole grains, and small, frequent feedings are easier on your digestion and cardiovascular system.

Daily aerobic exercise strengthens your heart and arteries and slows your basal heart rate, though it won't affect the rhythm.

Herbal and Folk Remedies

THE BERRIES and flowers of the hawthorn bush are said to normalize heart action and help calm palpitations. Tranquilizing herbs such as lemon balm, hops, passionflower, skullcap, and valerian may help if palpitations are caused by nervous stress.

Stroke

A stroke occurs when a blood vessel in the brain either breaks, bleeding into or onto the brain, or is suddenly blocked, producing paralysis and unconsciousness. The stroke can be the result of high blood pressure or arteriosclerosis, or of a blood clot or particles of tissue from the neck moving into the head.

Prevention is much the same as for high blood pressure: gentle exercise such as Yoga; massage therapy; a low- or no-fat diet, with lots of fiber and omega 3 oils; learning to avoid or manage stress; no smoking, and easy on the alcohol.

According to a Belgian study, people who take in a great deal of beta carotene recover more quickly from stroke.

Niacin (part of the B complex) supplements may help lower cholesterol. Researchers have found, however, that too much of this vitamin can lead to hepatitis and other liver disorders. When you need to take a B vitamin supplement, it is better to take the entire B complex. Foods rich in B vitamins include wheat germ, brewer's yeast, rice polish, and sunflower seeds.

If you take anti-clotting medication to help prevent stroke, the effects of the drugs can be counteracted by large amounts of broccoli, Dr. Sanford J. Kempin explained in a letter to the *New England Journal of Medicine*. Both broccoli and turnip greens are high in vitamin K, which promotes clotting. An average half-cup serving shouldn't be a problem, but you might want to consult your doctor.

Herbal and Folk Remedies

ACCORDING TO *Organic Gardening* magazine, a cup of peppermint tea a day can reduce the possibility of stroke by 40 percent. Aikira Suzuki and colleagues at the Saitama Institute of Public Health in Japan report that peppermint tea is an excellent source of potassium, having several times the amount found in an average banana.

Varicose Veins

Varicose veins are swollen or twisted blood vessels. Those in the rectum are called hemorrhoids, or piles. They are caused by a breakdown of the valves that keep the column of blood returning to your heart from settling in your veins. Genetic predisposition, prolonged standing, carrying extra weight, and pregnancy are possible causes.

Coping with varicose veins
*Advice from Ann Darlington, nurse-midwife at the Virginia Mason
Medical Center's Nurse-Midwifery Service in Seattle, Washington:*

During pregnancy you have a 50 percent increase in blood volume, and pregnancy hormones make varicose veins more capable of being distended. The problem will improve after delivery, but varicosities usually worsen with each pregnancy. Your veins are like a crooked river. During pregnancy, your blood vessels can become tortuous. Flow slows down at curves in the stream, further stretching the vessels. Veins have only one-way valves and no pulsation (as the arteries have), making it difficult for blood to reach those valves if flow and pressure are diminished.

- Exercise improves circulation; isometrics are especially good for pregnant women—they help the flow move upward, valve by valve.

- To counteract the force of gravity, wear thigh-high support hose and take frequent breaks to sit or lie with your feet higher than your heart.

- If a varicosity comes on suddenly, see your health care professional immediately, especially if the area around the vein is reddened. Don't rub the vein—you could dislodge a blood clot.

- Immersing yourself in cool water helps reduce varicosities and edema: the hydrostatic pressure from outside water helps "push" the edema's water back into your veins, and may help prevent overdistension of your veins. (Hot water causes flushing, which is increased flow to the skin as your body attempts to cool off.)

Naturopathic physician Lucy Smith at the Natural Health Clinic of Bastyr University in Seattle, Washington, recommends Vitamin E, which is very beneficial to your blood vessels and may help prevent varicosities.

Exercise can improve your circulation. Don't stand still. When you contract the muscles around your veins, you keep your blood moving—even moving your foot does it.

Herbal and Folk Remedies

COLD WITCH hazel compresses help constrict the veins temporarily, bringing relief.

HERBALIST JETHRO Kloss, in *Back to Eden,* recommends bathing the affected area frequently with strong oak bark tea, which is astringent, keeping your colon clear of wastes, and "purifying" your blood with an infusion made with one teaspoonful goldenseal, $1/2$ teaspoonful myrrh, and one pint water.

The Respiratory System:

From Asthma to Sore Throat

Of all your bodily systems, the respiratory is the one most immediately affected by your environment. With each breath you take, oxygen flows into your lungs, from whence it is transported to your bloodstream and cells. In your lungs are tiny air sacs where the exchange of oxygen and carbon dioxide takes place; there's also a network of tubes, descending in size from your windpipe to the minute bronchioles inside your lungs.

When there is mucus in your lungs, or your bronchial tissue becomes inflamed and swollen in response to infection or allergy, you experience breathing difficulties. Whether or not you will develop a breathing disorder is mostly determined by your genes, but your habits and your environment have much to do with how healthy your lungs will be.

Fresh air is essential. Even people who live in smoggy cities or industrial areas can control their indoor environment to some extent by keeping it smoke-free and supplied with an abundance of live, oxygen-releasing houseplants. Spider plants are said to be especially good at reducing indoor air pollution. Regular aerobic exercise, outdoors whenever possible, increases your lung capacity and the amount of oxygen you take in.

You can also choose not to smoke. Not only does smoking paralyze the cilia (tiny, hairlike structures that sweep your respiratory tract free of contaminants), it compromises your immune system, making you vulnerable to colds and flu. Smoking and inhaling tobacco smoke is the leading cause of a host of chronic and sometimes life-threatening diseases such as chronic bronchitis, emphysema, and lung cancer. Smoking cessation programs abound. Some, including twelve-step programs, are free except for a voluntary donation; others, such as those sponsored by the American Lung Association, are moderately priced.

Wendy Iseman, Communications Director for the American Lung Association of Brooklyn, New York, says that mucus, produced by goblet cells, is essential for cleansing the respiratory system, but too much can clog your lungs, making you wheeze and cough. Because mucus is sticky, it is also a breeding place for germs. Normal mucus is transparent, white, or gray, Iseman notes. Yellow or green mucus indicates an infection.

Ironically, in autumn, when the flu and cold season begins, we tend to eat more mucus-producing foods such as meat, eggs, starches, and dairy products. Many people with respiratory problems, and some health care professionals, believe that giving up dairy products reduces mucus production. If you are considering a dairy-free diet, see the list of alternative sources of calcium listed under OSTEOPOROSIS on page 140.

Asthma

Harvard Women's Health Watch reports that women are admitted to the hospital for asthma three times more often than men; the sufferer is more likely to be black than Caucasian. In her talks to parents in Brooklyn, Ms. Iseman has noted an especially high rate of asthma among Hispanics from Puerto Rico. The death rate from this disease has been rising since the end of the 1970s. Increased air pollution is a major factor; improper use of medication has also been cited.

The wheezing, coughing, and breathlessness of an asthma attack result from spasms of the bronchial muscles that constrict the airways and from inflammation of the airways. Harvard Women's Health Watch reports that a 1986 study found that 80 percent of women with asthma had abnormal levels of the hormones estradiol, progesterone, or cortisol.

Some allergens can trigger asthma. Harvard Women's Health Watch warns that vacuuming disrupts dust and keeps it airborne. They advise a double-filtered vacuum cleaner and special impermeable vacuum bags if you must vacuum. Other recommendations include using synthetic fiber rather than leather in your furnishings and foam rather than feather pillows in your bedroom. Also, avoid skin and hair preparations that contain vegetable gums or cottonseed or flaxseed extract; and be aware that aspirin and ibuprofen are allergens for some people. Other triggers for asthma can be air that is cold and dry or unusually damp, an upper respiratory infection, or stress.

Some people struggle daily with the disease, others have only an occasional episode every few years. Coughing, wheezing, shortness of breath, and a feeling of tightness in your chest are common symptoms of asthma. See your doctor if any of these symptoms persist for more than a week or two.

The National Heart, Lung and Blood Institute warns that asthma control is especially important during pregnancy, when your symptoms may become more severe, particularly between the twenty-ninth and thirty-sixth weeks. Uncontrolled asthma can lead to pregnancy complications or impair the development of the fetus.

Wendy Iseman of the American Lung Association of Brooklyn has these tips for asthma sufferers:

- Keep your home and—if possible—your workplace smoke-free. Woodsmoke from a fireplace or woodstove and tobacco smoke are irritants that can make your asthma worse.

- Smoking exacerbates asthma. So does drinking alcohol, which depresses breathing. Don't mix alcohol with medication.

- Asthma triggers, or causes, are varied and often unknown to the asthmatic. Some people have an allergic response to eggs, peanuts, nuts, strawberries, soybeans, chocolate, apples, orange juice, fish, or milk.

Other common allergens include dust, feathers, animal dander, dust mites, molds, pollens, industrial pollutants, cigarette and wood smoke, and perfumes; wood, vegetable, or metal dusts; chemicals, enzymes, and foods preserved with sulfites or seasoned with MSG.

- Keep an asthma diary to identify your triggers. In a small notebook that you can carry in your pocket or purse, write down everything that happens when you have asthma symptoms. List the date, time of day, and where you experienced breathing difficulties. For example, were you driving in heavy traffic, cleaning house, or feeling anger or other strong emotions? List any allergens you may have eaten or inhaled. Note whether you practiced self-care, and if you needed treatment in the hospital. Write down any medication(s) you took and possible side effects. This information is very helpful to take along on your regular clinic or doctor visits or if you should end up in the emergency room.

- If you are prone to asthma, try to avoid colds and flu by using some of the preventative measures described on page 100. Get flu and pneumonia shots. If you do get sick, take good care of yourself so your cold or flu won't lead to asthma.

- To protect your lungs from winter cold, cover your mouth with a scarf or wear a face mask.

- Remain indoors if possible when ozone or pollen levels are high.

- At home, avoid extremes of temperature and moisture level. If the air is too dry, keep a container of water on your stove or radiator. If you use a humidifier or a dehumidifier, discourage bacteria and mold by cleaning the device thoroughly twice a week.

- Air conditioning allows you to close the windows against pollen and mold spores. It also lowers humidity, which keeps down molds and dust mites indoors. Be sure to clean the filters at least once a week.

- Clean with a water and bleach solution to discourage mold, a frequent cause of asthma. Houseplant soil tends to harbor mold, so check it frequently or set your plants outdoors.

- Keep your bedroom as dust-free as possible. Remove all carpeting from the bedroom; use linoleum or bare wood flooring instead. At least once a week, damp-mop the floors with a solution of Murphy oil soap or other vegetable cleaning solution. Wash throw rugs, blankets, bedding, and curtains in very hot water if possible. Remove stuffed animals, venetian blinds, heavy curtains, and other dust catchers that can't be cleaned regularly. A window shade, cleaned regularly, may be an alternative.

- As many as 75 percent of asthma patients are allergic to dust mites, specifically their droppings. These microscopic organisms are probably the motes you see when you shake out your bedclothing. They live in carpets and bedclothes, feeding on tiny flakes of shedded human skin. Wrap your pillows and mattress in plastic casing to keep them free of dust and dust mites. Wash all bed linens in hot water to kill the mites.

- The droppings or crumbled corpses of cockroaches, which can get into house dust, are also highly allergenic. This dust can make your eyes run or give you an ear infection.

- Dogs and cats are a big problem with asthma because many people are allergic to their dander. If you can't get rid of your pets, at least keep them out of your bedroom, give them a bath once a week, and vacuum frequently.

- Don't wear perfume or use aerosol sprays or strong-smelling chemicals in your home.

- Many people suffer nighttime asthma attacks. Mucus collects when you lie down flat, so prop yourself on pillows to prevent this from happening.

- Take your medication as prescribed. If your medication doesn't seem to be helping you, don't decide on your own to give it up—consult with your doctor.

- Increase your lung capacity with exercise such as walking, swimming, or karate. If exercising makes you cough, take your medication beforehand. Pollen and pollution are lowest early in the day, so that's the best time to exercise.

- Drink lots of water—it helps thin the mucus so it can be easily expelled.

- Ask your doctor for a peak flow meter and instructions on how to use it. This tubular plastic device measures the volume of air passing out of your lungs. Using it every morning helps you avoid emergencies. Since an asthma attack can take days to develop, you can tell by the air volume reading on your peak flow meter whether obstruction in your lungs is building up. When your reading is low, take your medication or, if indicated, call your doctor or go to the emergency room.

The *European Journal of Respiration* reported in 1984 that in a Swedish study a low-tryptophan diet produced fewer asthma symptoms. Tryptophan is a precursor to serotonin, a blood vessel constrictor stored in blood platelets. Serotonin is linked with asthma attacks. High-tryptophan foods include carrots, beets, celery, spinach, alfalfa, turkey, and milk.

Stephen Hoffman, M.D., writes in the *Harvard Health Letter* that a typical night attack possibly occurs as a result of stomach acid that flows back into the esophagus and stimulates the vagus (a major nerve to the lungs) to signal the bronchi to constrict. It may help to change your eating patterns—try big meals early in the day and a light supper, or several small meals a day.

In India, Yoga centers have treated asthma victims for more than fifty years by teaching meditation, breathing exercises, and postures that tone the thoraxic and abdominal muscles and reduce stress.

Exercising to increase lung capacity may help lessen the frequency or severity of attacks. Patients who practice deep-breathing exercises also experience significant improvement. For example, place your hands on your stomach between your ribs and navel as you stand, sit, or recline. Feel your diaphragm, moving it in and out against your hands. Inhale to a count of four, exhale to a count of eight, gradually increasing the count to increase lung capacity and strengthen your diaphragm.

When you are short of breath, the American Lung Association of Brooklyn recommends pursed-lip breathing: (1) Relax. Let your neck and shoulders droop. (2) Breathe in slowly. (3) Purse your lips in a whistling position, and blow out slowly and evenly. Try to take at least twice as long blowing out as you did breathing in. (4) Relax. Repeat the pursed-lip breathing until you no longer feel breathless. If you get dizzy, rest for a few breaths.

Herbal and Folk Remedies

CAFFEINE IS a potent bronchodilator. To subdue an acute asthma attack, drink three six-ounce cups of lukewarm or cool coffee or six cups of tea. Caribbean people boil cocoa (cacao) beans, also a source of caffeine, for the same purpose. **Warning:** Chocolate is a common allergen; be sure it isn't one of yours. Asthmatic coffee drinkers will no doubt be pleased to hear that indulging their habit in moderation can actually be helpful in reducing symptoms. According to an Italian study, people who drink three or more cups of coffee a day have fewer bronchial asthma attacks.

IF YOU are allergic to pollen, a daily cup of chamomile tea or a tablespoonful of honey that was gathered within a ten-mile radius of your home may desensitize you to this allergen and immunize you for the allergy season. **Warning:** If you are allergic to ragweed, which is botanically related to chamomile, take only a tablespoon or so of the tea at first and gradually work up to a cup.

GARLIC, A popular folk remedy for respiratory and vascular ailments, has been the subject of several laboratory studies. Researchers have found that eating garlic sauteed in oil increases your production of vinyldithins, which are bronchial relaxers.

TWO CARIBBEAN recipes: (1) Two tablespoons olive oil, one tablespoon minced raw garlic, and a dash of honey. (2) Mix equal portions of minced

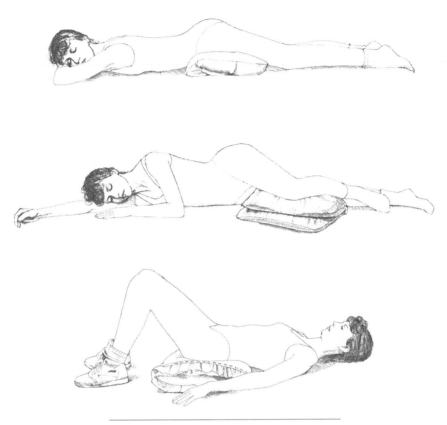

To drain mucus from your lungs, the American Lung Association of Brooklyn advises clearing your lungs at least twice a day (check with your doctor first). The best times are before breakfast and an hour before sleep. Lie in one of the positions illustrated above and practice pursed-lip breathing to open your passageways. When you feel like coughing, cough twice—once to loosen mucus, then again to bring it up. Don't swallow the mucus.

raw red onion, honey, and lemon. Take one or two teaspoonfuls of either potion in the morning and evening.

MANY RURAL people believe that chewing honeycomb helps them recover from an attack.

FOR MORE than five thousand years, the seeds and fan-shaped leaves of the ginkgo tree have been used in China for asthma and other disorders. The seeds are boiled to make a decoction that dries up mucus in the lungs. You can also steep a teaspoonful of the leaves in boiling water for ten minutes, or take a few drops of the extract—both are sold in health food and herbal outlets.

Colds and Flu

Probably no ailment has as many folk remedies as the common cold, and there are almost as many for the common flu. According to the American Lung Association, more than one hundred viruses cause colds. Antibiotics, which combat bacteria, are ineffective against the viruses that cause colds and flu; over-the-counter preparations offer only temporary relief and often have adverse side effects.

Influenza viruses appear to be airborne. When exposed to these viruses, your immune cells produce free radicals that result in flu symptoms. Women seem to be more susceptible than men. Stress increases your susceptibility. A simple cold or bout with the flu is not serious—most people recover from a cold in a week or ten days, from flu in twice that time. However, neglecting a cold or flu can make you vulnerable to secondary infections, so if you have asthma, emphysema, or other chronic lung disease, be sure to consult your doctor.

Hints on avoiding colds from Wendy Iseman
of the American Lung Association of Brooklyn:

- Cold viruses live in your throat year round and flare up in wintertime when artificial heating dries your mucus passages. To avoid the dry air that is unhealthy for your respiratory system, replenish moisture with a humidifier or set containers of water on the stove or radiators.

- Although some cold viruses are airborne, most are transmitted by hand; for example, when you touch a germ-laden doorknob or telephone or shake hands with someone who has a cold, then touch your eyes, nose, or mouth. A good preventative is to wash your hands thoroughly with soap and water a minimum of five times a day. To avoid spreading a cold, as soon as you blow your nose, put the used tissue in a closed receptacle such as a paper or plastic bag and wash your hands afterward.

- Drink lots of water to thin mucus so it is easier to expel.

- Avoid smoking, which paralyzes the hairlike cells in your nasal passages that keep them clean. Limit your intake of alcohol, which weakens your respiratory system.

Herbal and Folk Remedies

···

ACCORDING TO Dr. Andrew Weil, holistic physician and author of *Spontaneous Healing*, inhaling pesticides, herbicides, solvents, or chemicals with strong odors can drain your immunity. Strengthening your immune system helps you resist virus-induced disorders. The best-known immunizer is echinacea. Take ½ teaspoon infused in boiling water or the equivalent in capsules once a day every other week. Other immunizers include the Chinese herb astragalus; oyster, shiitake, enokidake, and maitake mushrooms; tea made from the root of the Chinese mushroom zhuling; St. John's wort; zinc, selenium, beta carotene, and vitamins A, B, C, and E.

MEGADOSES OF vitamin C—up to 1,000 milligrams—help some people ward off colds and flu. People who tend to form kidney stones or have kidney disease are not advised to take such megadoses.

GARLIC IS a centuries-old Mediterranean remedy that has become universal. A Provo, Utah, study showed that raw garlic kills nearly 100 percent of rhinoviruses. Keeping a fresh clove of garlic between your cheeks and teeth to prevent a cold from developing is acceptable in some cultures. Otherwise, chop a raw clove finely and swallow it at bedtime. A few sprigs of fresh parsley help deodorize your breath.

ACCORDING TO D. C. Jarvis, a Vermont family practitioner who wrote about folk medicine in the 1950s, vinegar and honey, which supposedly restore the body's acid balance, may also head off a cold. For the first day or two when you have cold symptoms, take a tablespoonful of each in a glass of hot water with a pinch of cayenne pepper every two hours while you're awake. Bundle up warmly—the cayenne helps you sweat out toxins.

TRADITIONAL CHINESE medicine prescribes warming herbs and spices to be taken at the first sign of a cold. Ginger is most often recommended. Boil a walnut–sized gingerroot, cinnamon stick, ½ teaspoon cloves, and a teaspoon coriander seed in a pint of water for about 30 minutes. When you take the mixture from the fire, add a teaspoon each of lemon juice and honey. Ginseng, a panacea in China and other Asian countries, is also taken to build resistance to colds.

JAMAICANS BOIL an entire cerasee plant, seeds and all, for twenty to thirty minutes, then drink the broth when a cold is coming on.

SCOTS, NEW ENGLANDERS, and thousands of other folks swear by a bedtime hot toddy made by pouring a cup of boiling water over one tablespoon each sugar, lemon and whiskey.

SCOTLAND'S SHETLAND Islanders take PIRR when they feel a chill: 2 tablespoons oatmeal, 1 teaspoon sugar, $1/2$ teaspoon cream of tartar, a dash of milk, and 1 cup water. Mix the oatmeal, sugar, and cream of tartar in a warm jug or thermos, add enough milk to make a smooth paste, then pour boiling water over the mixture, stirring all the time. Take piping hot before retiring.

FOOD WRITER Mike Moore reported in a *New York Times* article that the fresh grated taproot of horseradish has been used since antiquity for its warming qualities. Modern researchers have discovered that the root is antibiotic, helping fight bacterial infections, and rich in vitamin C.

INHALING STEAM at the first sign of a cold is an ancient and universal strategy. The *Journal of the American Medical Association* reports that a twenty-minute exposure to heated, humidified air increases the temperature of the nasal passages enough so that "viral replication would cease," resulting in an 80 percent reduction of rhinoviruses within a day. Throw a handful of peppermint, sage, chamomile, eucalyptus, or wintergreen in a pot of boiling water. Turn off the heat, drape a towel over your head, and inhale. This may kill nasal viruses and break up sinus and lung congestion.

RUSSIANS AND other Eastern and Northern Europeans take saunas to ward off colds and flu. The hot steam may kill rhinoviruses and certainly will induce perspiration, which helps you throw off toxins. This method is not used after the cold is established.

IF YOU do catch cold, don't suppress sweating, vomiting, or diarrhea, which gets rid of toxins. Dr. Lucy Smith, Naturopathic physician at the Natural Health Clinic of Bastyr University in Seattle, Washington, recommends this naturopathic treatment, which mimics the healing effects of fever by heating your body: after a twenty-minute soak in a hot tub, drink hot ginger tea, adding honey and lemon if desired; bundle up in socks, cap, and sweatsuit or flannel pajamas; climb into bed with extra blankets, tucking a small pillow under your knees. Stay in bed for at least an hour; overnight is fine.

ANOTHER NATUROPATHIC treatment is to stimulate an immune response by heating, cooling, then reheating your body. Soak in a hot tub for twenty minutes, then wet a pair of thin cotton ankle socks in cold water, wring them out, put them on, add a pair of heavy wool socks, and get into bed. However, don't use this treatment if you have chronic cold feet. When you have finished a sweat treatment, bathe or sponge off so the toxins your body eliminated won't be reabsorbed.

RUSSIANS DRINK hot tea with strawberry jam or vodka, whiskey, or tequila, spiked with pepper, and get into bed wearing a T-shirt under nightwear and socks. Some Russians rub themselves all over with vodka first.

ANOTHER RUSSIAN remedy is to soak in a hot bath, then drink a cup of hot milk with honey or butter and a pinch of baking soda. An alternative recipe is hot milk with one teaspoon each honey and butter and a dash of mineral water. Drink the mixture as hot as possible before getting into bed.

TO STIMULATE perspiration, Jamaicans boil a crushed fresh gingerroot for twenty-five to thirty minutes and drink the broth. Fevergrass tea, made from a Caribbean herb, is used for the same purpose.

SCOTTISH TREACLE TOFFEE contains ingredients that are warming, and helps you sweat, especially if you bundle up after eating one or two. You'll need 2 pounds sugar, 1 pound black molasses, ¼ pound butter, and a pinch of black pepper. Melt the butter and molasses, add the sugar and pepper, and stir over low heat for 20 minutes. When the mixture has cooked to the hard-ball stage, remove from the heat and pour on a cookie sheet. When cool enough to handle, roll into balls of the desired size, wrap in waxed paper, and store in airtight container. **Note:** instead of pepper, add 2 teaspoons powdered ginger with the sugar.

OATMEAL BROSE is another Scottish remedy taken hot at bedtime. To make it, pour 2 cups of boiling water over a handful steel-cut oats, 1 tablespoon each sugar and butter, and a pinch of salt, stirring all the while. Let the mixture settle a minute, then sip the broth off the top—don't eat the oatmeal.

A HOT BATH with aromatic herbs added is a traditional remedy for the aches and pains of colds and flu. The American Botanical Council/Herb

Research Foundation reports that research at Kiev Institute of Physiology shows that several minutes after sweating, your pores stay open and absorb any solution from the skin surface—hence the effect of herbal baths. Pine needle baths are said to increase production of white blood cells, which fight infection.

IN THE CARIBBEAN, traditional remedies include swallowing eucalyptus pills and rubbing the oil on the skin.

Cough, Chest Congestion, and Bronchitis

Most coughs are an attempt to expel mucus from your lungs. Expectorants thin the mucus so it can be expelled more easily. The Public Citizen Health Research Group says the best expectorant is water. Drink at least eight glasses a day.

Hot pepper helps clear congestion. Jean Carper, author of *Food: Your Miracle Medicine* and other books on nutrition, recommends twenty drops Tabasco sauce in a glass of tomato juice.

Homemade Chicken Soup: The Classic Cold Remedy

Laboratory studies reveal that chicken soup contains ingredients that may reduce the body's inflammation response, as well as the amino acid acetyl cysteine, which thins mucus in the lungs. Some ingredients in the following soup recipe thin mucus; others induce perspiration, build resistance, or are antiseptic. The allicin in garlic, a germ killer *par excellence,* also thins mucus.

To 3 cups chicken stock add 4 garlic cloves, 5 or 6 fresh basil leaves, 1 tablespoon fresh or $1^{1}/_{2}$ teaspoons of each of these dried herbs: dillweed, thyme, parsley, marjoram, chervil, a pinch of cayenne pepper, and two or three slices fresh or $1^{1}/_{2}$ teaspoons dried gingerroot. Eat a bowlful as hot as possible at least once a day, preferably at bedtime.

Herbal and Folk Remedies

··

IN CALIFORNIA and the Caribbean, where the herb yerba santa grows, two or three leaves are steeped in a cup of boiling water. Take a tablespoonful at a time; at bedtime sip a half cup. Yerba buena, also a Caribbean herb, can be used instead. Look for these herbs in your health food or herb store.

YOU CAN make a Puerto Rican cough syrup with the juice of 2 lemons, $^1/_2$ ounce honey, 2 cups whiskey or other hard liquor, and 2 pieces of fresh anise or 2 teaspoons anise seed. Boil for 10 minutes and take by the teaspoonful as needed.

IN JAMAICA, whooping cough is treated with a potion made by boiling together 1 ginger root, 2 cloves garlic, and 2 cups water for 15 minutes. Take by the teaspoonful as needed.

AMERICAN INDIANS roasted onions, and when they were soft, they squeezed out the juice and mixed it with red clover syrup and honey. The Indians also boiled the onions and made a kind of porridge with them as a cold preventative.

GRATE A CLOVE or two of garlic and mix with a teaspoonful of honey; take as needed.

SCOTTISH ONION COUGH CURE: Slice 1 large onion into an ovenproof bowl, add 1 cup sugar, $^1/_2$ cup lemon juice, and a dash of cinnamon. Bake in a preheated oven at 300°F. for about 2 hours, or until the sugar is melted and the onion soft. Remove the onion and sip the juice.

IN THE SCOTTISH HEBRIDES, people gather carageen seaweed in rock pools, then wash and dry it for a variety of uses. (You may be able to gather your own if you live in a coastal area; otherwise, you'll find it in health food stores.) The iodine and sulfur it contains are often recommended for chest troubles. CARAGEEN MOLD: $^1/_2$ ounce dried carageen, $1^1/_2$ pints milk, 1 beaten egg (optional), sugar to taste, flavoring. Wash the carageen and steep in cold water for 20 minutes; drain, and place in a saucepan. Add the milk, bring slowly to a boil, and simmer until thickened. Strain, add the egg, if desired, then the sugar and flavor with lemon, orange juice or sherry to taste. An alternate flavoring method is to simmer with bay leaf, lemon peel, dried elder flowers, or cinnamon stick. Pour into a mold and chill until set.

SCOTTISH DRAMBUIE COUGH CURE: mix 2 tablespoons Drambuie with 4 tablespoons honey, shake well, and use as a cough syrup. **Warning:** Don't use Drambuie if you are pregnant or have a problem with alcohol.

RICHARD LUCAS, in his book *Nature's Medicines,* published in the 1960s, recounts a remedy used successfully by a London physician for many years to treat children with whooping cough: Chop several cloves of garlic fine, lay on a cloth, and apply to the soles of your feet with the cloth against the skin; the garlic layer should be about $1/4$ inch thick. To prevent blistering or irritation, first grease the soles of your feet with petroleum jelly. Cover the layer of garlic with another cloth and secure to your feet with a pair of old socks. Leave the garlic on overnight. Lucus advises that any night cough can be treated in this way.

THIS VERMONT folk remedy was recorded years ago by Dr. D. C. Jarvis in his book *Folk Medicine.* It works on the most stubborn coughs. Boil a whole lemon for 10 minutes. When it is cool enough to handle, roll the lemon back and forth on a hard surface, then cut in half and squeeze it into a pint of raw honey. Add a teaspoon glycerin and take as often as needed.

Dry Coughs

The tickling and irritation that can follow a sore throat may cause a dry cough. Honey is moisturizing and soothes your mucous membranes; syrups and cough drops also help soothe your throat and keep it moist.

Tea made with red clover, wild cherry bark, licorice root, or slippery elm bark and sweetened with honey helps soothe a dry cough.

Some Russian Remedies for Dry Cough

Black tea with lemon and honey, fresh raspberries, or raspberry preserve.

Milk and honey.

Warm milk with a fig boiled in it.

One tablespoon honey dissolved in a glass of boiling water.

Hollow out a black radish and fill the cavity with a teaspoon of honey. After two or three hours, drink the juice.

Herbal and Folk Remedies for Bronchial Congestion:

MUSTARD PLASTERS were an official remedy in the U.S. Pharmacopoeia early in this century. Naturopaths still prescribe them to loosen up a dry cough or tight chest and stimulate the lungs to expectorate. Mix a tablespoon or two of dry mustard with a cup of flour. Add hot water to make a paste, then spread the paste over a thin cloth. Place the cloth on your chest, add a second layer of cloth, then a layer of plastic, and a heating pad or hot water bottle on top. Don't leave the plaster on for more than fifteen or twenty minutes, and check frequently to make sure your skin is not irritated. To avoid irritation or blistering, remove the mustard plaster immediately if your skin is painful and glowing red.

GINGER, WHICH is warming, has a similar effect. Boil a piece of a ginger root for about twenty minutes, soak a cloth in the tea, and place on your chest. Keep the compress warm by covering it with a layer of plastic and a towel.

NATUROPATH DR. Lucy Smith recommends a castor oil pack, which is used by naturopaths to draw out infection and congestion. To prepare a castor oil pack, put two to four thicknesses of flannel cloth in a large ovenproof pan; saturate the cloth with castor oil, and warm the compress in the oven for ten minutes or so. Wring out the cloth so it is damp but not dripping, lay it on your chest, and keep it warm with a layer of plastic and a hot water bottle or heating pad.

TO RELIEVE chest pain caused by congestion, Russians mash a potato that has been boiled or baked in its jacket, spread the potato on a cotton cloth, roll the whole thing in a towel, and place on the chest. To keep the potato warm, cover with a layer of plastic or waxed paper. Leave on for at least five hours, preferably overnight. Cupping is also used in Russia for dealing with chest congestion.

OTHER DECONGESTANTS include hot, steamy showers and hot tea made with peppermint, rosemary, or thyme to break up congestion. Hot chili peppers, Chinese mustard, or other spicy foods also loosen mucus.

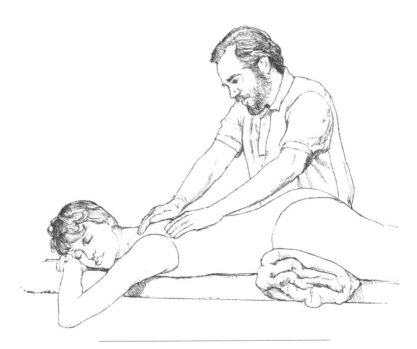

THE AMERICAN LUNG ASSOCIATION OF BROOKLYN RECOMMENDS THIS METHOD OF CLAPPING OR VIBRATING THE CHEST WITH CUPPED HANDS TO LOOSEN MUCUS SO IT CAN BE EXPECTORATED.

Fever

Heat is nature's way of killing off disease organisms, so don't suppress a fever unless it is very high. Instead, encourage perspiration with hot baths and hot drinks made with sweat-inducing herbs (see HERBAL AND FOLK REMEDIES, below). The evaporation of moisture on your skin will gradually reduce your temperature.

Herbal and Folk Remedies

HERBAL TEAS that stimulate perspiration include warm elder or linden blossoms, hot boneset tea sweetened with honey, and peppermint, hyssop, lilac, yarrow, or the bark of cinnamon, pine, spruce or hemlock.

HIGH OR persistent fever can be brought down with salicylate-containing herbs such as willow, meadowsweet, and wintergreen. Peruvian bark (cinchona), which contains quinine, excels at bringing down a fever. **Warning:** Don't take quinine if you are pregnant because it stimulates uterine contractions.

ONE RUSSIAN remedy is to sponge the skin with vodka, red wine, or cider vinegar and fan the damp skin to bring down a fever. Another is to sponge the skin with a solution of one part vinegar and two parts water, then wet a cloth with the mixture and place it on the forehead. The cloth is dipped in the solution periodically to keep it wet. Russians and other Eastern Europeans also sip tea made with one teaspoon black tea and one teaspoon rose hips or black currants and honey to sweeten.

IN THE Caribbean, aloe is placed on the forehead, the soles of the feet, and all body openings. A Caribbean brew to stimulate perspiration calls for 3 cinnamon sticks, ¼ cup anise, ½ cup sugar, and 2 cups water. Boil for 10 minutes and sip hot as needed.

IN AFRICA, three mango leaves or an unspecified number of eucalyptus leaves are boiled in a cup of water and sipped hot with sugar three times a day.

Rhinitis
(Congested, Runny Nose)

Your nasal membrane responds to allergens and viruses by releasing histamine, a chemical that causes your nasal membranes to swell and release excess mucus. Yellow or green nasal mucus indicates a bacterial infection that should be treated by your doctor.

Some medical experts believe that mucus flowing from your nose gets rid of toxins and corrects inflammation. Preparations that dry up secretions can cause blocked air passages and coughing.

Coping with a runny nose and nasal congestion
Advice from Melissa Pashcow, M.D., associate attending in the Department of Otolaryngology at New York Eye and Ear Infirmary and clinical instructor in Otolaryngology at New York Medical College:

- To help relieve chronic nasal conditions, douche your nasal tract with Alkalol, an herbal preparation available at pharmacies. This is applied using a nasal douche cup.

- Humidifiers and vaporizers help relieve nasal congestion. However, because of the moisture they generate, they breed germs. Be sure to clean your humidifier regularly and use distilled water. Chlorinated or softened water or water with a high mineral content can irritate your sensitive mucous membranes.

- A hot, steamy shower is an excellent decongestant. Your nose is your body's humidifier. Nasal blood vessels swell and give off heat and moisture, which in turn warm and moisturize the air that enters your respiratory system. The steamy shower takes over the work of humidifying, allowing the blood vessels in your nose to constrict and your breathing passages to open.

- Leaning over a bowl of steaming water—another old-fashioned cold remedy—similarly warms the inside of your nose, so the blood vessels won't have to swell to warm the air, allowing your nose to decongest.

The American Academy of Otolaryngology warns that nasal blood vessels that are persistently dilated can lose their capacity to constrict. They become somewhat like varicose veins, filling up when you lie down to sleep. If this happens, the academy recommends sleeping with the head of your bed elevated two to four inches.

Here are a few of the teas sipped around the world to combat colds and flu:

- A Scottish bedtime potion is two tablespoons black currant jam dissolved in $1\frac{1}{2}$ cups boiling water.

- In Poland and other Eastern European nations, the teas of choice are linden (lime blossom) with honey and chamomile with baked garlic.

- In South America and the Caribbean, cold sufferers drink yerba maté, a popular herbal tea, available in the United States at most tea and herb suppliers.

- Licorice or horsetail tea is said to relieve a runny nose.

- Chinese ephedra, an herb sold in health food stores, contains ephedrine, an alkaloid used in pharmaceuticals for colds, asthma, and hay fever. Ephedrine constricts blood vessels and dries up mucus. **Warning:** Like most oral decongestants, the tea is very drying and raises your blood pressure temporarily. Drink no more than one cup of the tea every four hours, and don't take it at all if you have high blood pressure.

Herbal and Folk Remedies

OTOLARYNGOLOGIST DR. Melissa Pashcow notes that sipping hot tea, a popular folk remedy around the world, works mainly because of the steam, which acts as a nasal decongestant.

SNIFFING POWDERED vitamin C thins nasal mucus and helps get rid of a cold. Some health food and vitamin suppliers sell this item. You can also pulverize tablets.

A RUSSIAN strategy to kill rhinoviruses is to wash the inside of your nose with soap and water.

LELORD KORDEL, writing on folk medicine, reports that an Eskimo remedy for stuffy nose is to pack it with snow. The cold, he explains, contracts the membranes and opens up the nasal passages. If you don't happen to have any snow around, he recommends that you snuff two cups cold water with a teaspoon each of bicarbonate of soda and Epsom salts added. **Warning:** Do this carefully so you won't suck water into your eustachian tubes.

Rhinitis, Allergic
(Hay Fever)

When an inhaled allergen contacts antibodies in your nose, the reaction releases histamine, a chemical that dilates your blood vessels, stimulates your mucus-producing glands, and inflames and congests the membranes lining your nasal air passages. The result is sneezing, runny nose, upper respiratory irritation and itching, and red, itchy, and/or swollen eyes.

Consulting an allergist is the quickest way to identify the allergens, but sometimes the answer is fairly obvious. The majority of hay fever sufferers are allergic to ragweed, which flourishes in late summer and early fall at about the same time as goldenrod is in bloom. Spring grass and tree pollens are also common allergens. If your symptoms appear at the same time every year, you can narrow down the possible sources.

Chronic hay fever may be caused by household dust and dust mites, (microscopic insects related to spiders) that nourish themselves mainly on particles of sloughed human skin. Dust mite droppings are a common allergen. The preferred hangout of dust mites is your bed, where most shed skin accumulates. Experts recommend a dustproof mattress cover; pillows and blankets made of synthetic materials; banishing dust catchers such as carpeting and venetian blinds, and frequent and thorough housecleaning.

Mold is another year-round allergen. It grows everywhere outdoors, especially in humid climates. Indoors, it grows in houseplant soil and damp rooms such as basements and bathrooms. Air conditioning helps filter out molds and pollen from outdoors; a dehumidifier reduces damp and mold indoors. Both should be cleaned at least once a week.

Pets—or their dander—are other frequent offenders. If you must keep them, banish them from the bedroom and vacuum frequently.

Food allergies are not always so easy to identify. You could try eliminating certain foods, one at a time, that you suspect to see if your symptoms improve. Some people are allergic to food additives. Reading food labels is a very useful habit.

For more information on allergies, see ASTHMA on pages 94–99.

Herbal and Folk Remedies

A DAILY cup or two of chamomile tea or tablespoonful of honey gathered from within a ten-mile radius of where you live may immunize you by the time hay fever season rolls around. If you are allergic to ragweed, begin with only a few teaspoons of chamomile, a botanical relative, then work up to a cup or more.

Sinus Infections

Sinusitis is an inflammation of the mucous membrane lining your sinuses (cavities within your skull that drain into your nose). When the membrane becomes inflamed, it swells up, blocking your sinus openings, so the cavities cannot drain. The blockage can lead to infection, fever, and severe headaches. None of the self-care measures listed below are a substitute for medical evaluation and treatment.

A sinus infection can be a complication of cold or flu, so the best way to avoid one is to take care of the initial respiratory infection.

Allergy is a factor in some sinusitis. You may find it helpful to identify allergens so you can avoid them.

Some health professionals believe that poor nutrition may be a factor in some sinus infections. A well-balanced diet with plenty of fresh fruits and vegetables is essential. Foods rich in vitamins E and C help build immunity; vitamin A helps protect your mucous membranes. Limit or eliminate mucus-producing dairy products, meats, starches, and eggs.

Cover your nose with a scarf when you go out into cold, dry air.

Otolaryngologist Dr. Melissa Pashcow recommends a hot compress laid over your cheeks for ten or fifteen minutes two or three times a day. The heat dilates your blood vessels and stimulates circulation.

Herbal and Folk Remedies

DRINK AT least eight glasses of water or other fluid to thin mucus, so it can be eliminated. Ginger, thyme, peppermint, and spearmint teas help loosen mucus.

VAPORIZERS RELIEVE congestion by taking over the humidifying work of your nose, thus allowing your nasal blood vessels and membranes to constrict. You can get the same effect from a hot, steamy shower or leaning over a pot of hot water with a towel draped over your head. A handful of peppermint or a few eucalyptus leaves in the water will boost the decongestant power of the steam.

BREATHE EASY or any herb tea containing Chinese ephedra helps shrink nasal membranes and allow mucus to drain. **Warning:** Don't take ephedra if you have hypertension—it temporarily raises the blood pressure.

EATING HORSERADISH, raw garlic, raw hot chili or other hot peppers, or Chinese mustard clears the sinuses, as aficionados of these foods have already discovered.

IN RUSSIAN folk medicine, heat is used to stimulate circulation and relieve pressure. Heat salt in a skillet, spread it on a cloth, and place it on the bridge of your nose. Heated flaxseed or even hot hard-boiled eggs are also used.

DISSOLVE A teaspoon salt in a cup boiling water. When the solution has cooled, snuff it up through your nostrils into your mouth. Repeat the procedure. **Warning:** This must be done very carefully so you won't suck the water into your eustachian tubes or lungs. Nasal douche cups, which have a spout designed to fit into the nostril, are sold in pharmacies. Some New Age stores or those that cater to Yoga practitioners also sell Neti pots designed to cleanse the nose.

Sore Throat

Inflammation of the mucous membranes of your throat and vocal cords causes irritation and sometimes hoarseness. Most sore throats are the result of an infection, but prolonged shouting, singing, public speaking, postnasal drip, or heartburn can cause sore throat and hoarseness.

Preventing and treating a sore throat—
Advice from Otolaryngologist Dr. Melissa Pashcow:

- To avoid an infectious sore throat, don't share soap, towels, or utensils with people who are infected. Wipe telephone receivers and earpieces with a small amount of alcohol (too much of any fluid can injure electronic equipment). If your immune system is suppressed, you may want to take extra precautions.

- The purpose of gargling is to dissolve mucus, cleanse your throat, and provide astringency. Back when I was in medical school, the old-timers introduced me to Alkalol, an herbal preparation sold in pharmacies. I continue to recommend a 50 percent dilution as a gargle.

- White spots inside your mouth and throat accompanied by chills and a fever indicate strep throat. This should never be neglected—see your doctor immediately.

- If you suddenly have difficulty swallowing, talking, or breathing, seek help at once. In some instances, an allergic reaction or infection can cause such severe inflammation and swelling that your windpipe is closed off.

Antihistamines dry your throat, and alcohol mouthwash irritates it. Smoking and inhaling secondhand smoke are also irritants.

Don't eat dairy products—they produce mucus, a breeding ground for bacteria.

Herbal and Folk Remedies

NATUROPATH DR. Lucy Smith recommends a carrot poultice. Grate a large carrot and spread it on cheesecloth or other thin material; wrap the cheesecloth around your throat and cover the poultice with a scarf. For

The late naturalist Euell Gibbons created this recipe for horehound lozenges, a traditional sore throat and cough remedy he describes in *Stalking the Wild Asparagus.*

Soak ¾ cup horehound (health food and herbal suppliers sell this herb) and ¼ cup fresh thyme in cold water overnight. Strain and squeeze all the juice from the leaves. Place the liquid and one cup honey in a saucepan and boil until the mixture forms a hard ball when dropped in cold water. Cool slightly, spread on an oiled baking sheet, and cut into half teaspoon-sized pieces before the mixture hardens. Store wrapped in waxed paper in an airtight container.

additional relief, apply either a cold compress made by adding crushed ice to the carrot, or a hot compress made by dipping the cloth and grated carrot in hot water.

AFRICANS DRINK carrot juice with a spoonful of sugar for colds, sore throat, and bronchitis. Carrots are rich in beta carotene, good for mucous membranes.

THE SIMPLEST sore throat remedy is to gargle four or five times a day with one teaspoon salt dissolved in eight ounces hot water. Some people add two drops iodine or a little honey. Dr. Melissa Pashcow warns against adding too much salt. A strong salt solution, she says, can be caustic and aggravate the pain.

AN EFFECTIVE gargle is soothing, astringent, and/or antiseptic. Some herbs that have at least one of these virtues are myrrh (astringent and antiseptic, very healing to cuts and abrasions, often recommended by herbalists for mouth and gum problems); horehound, sage, white pond lily root, and fennel (astringent); marshmallow root, psyllium seeds, Irish moss, and linseed (coats your throat, soothing, healing); chamomile and thyme (antiseptic; chamomile is also antiinflammatory).

GARGLE WITH one part peroxide to three parts water—it's antiseptic.

SUCK ON half a lemon soaked in salt water.

SUCK SLIPPERY elm lozenges to coat your throat.

THE FOLLOWING remedy was related by a young Russian, who claims it works for his family—probably because the exercise increases circulation. Stick out your tongue as far as you can, turn down your head, and keep your sore muscles extended for one minute, then massage your throat for a minute. Do this every thirty minutes during the day. The next day, he adds, maybe you will have no sore throat.

Laryngitis

Frequently the aftermath of a sore throat, laryngitis, or hoarseness, is an inflammation of the vocal cords. Contact with chemicals or other irritants or overuse of the voice can also cause laryngitis.

Treating laryngitis
Advice from Otolaryngologist Dr. Melissa Pashcow:

- It's best if you stay at home and rest your vocal cords as much as possible. If you must go out to work, communicate with a pad and paper. When you do speak, don't whisper—it tightens the muscles of your voice box, stressing your vocal cords more than does talking in a normal voice. To ease the strain on your throat, let the sound come from your diaphragm rather than your throat.

- Keep your throat moist with lozenges or chewing gum. Drink hot soups and liquids—inhaling the steam moisturizes and soothes your throat. Adding honey to your tea moisturizes, soothes, and coats your throat. Standing in a hot, steamy shower is also beneficial. Use a humidifier or vaporizer to keep the air moist.

- If you have difficulty swallowing or breathing, see your doctor right away. You should also see your doctor if your symptoms last more than two or three days.

Herbal and Folk Remedies

LICORICE TEA is soothing. Also, tea containing epinephrine constricts the blood vessels and reduces vocal cord swelling. The ephedrine in Chinese ephedra, an ingredient in Breathe Easy tea, sold in many supermarkets, has a similar effect. Do not use, however, if you have hypertension.

WHEN TRAVELING by plane, where the air is dry, be sure to take in plenty of fluids.

6

The Musculoskeletal System:

From Arthritis to Sports Injuries

We tend to think of our musculoskeletal system as mostly bones, the muscles that move them, and the joints that permit their flexibility. In fact, muscle is our most vulnerable and ubiquitous tissue, from the indispensable heart to the tiny muscles that line our blood vessels and the larger ones that line our intestines. Of all the organ systems in the human body, this one is most immediately affected by wear and tear, aging, poor nutrition, overexertion, recklessness, and the prevailing climate that surrounds us—in other words, by stress. It is also the system most jeopardized by inactivity—a fact that becomes more relevant the older we get.

Arthritis

According to the American College of Rheumatology, there are more than one hundred diseases that cause the joint swelling, pain, and loss of motion of arthritis. For so common a disease—most of us will have at least a touch of it if we live long enough—arthritis is surprisingly mysterious. To date, there is still no cure, and relatively little is known about its origins. Many arthritics can forecast rainy weather by joints that ache in response to increased barometric pressure. Some herbalists and other health practitioners believe that an excess of uric acid, which has already been linked to gout (a form of arthritis), may be a suspect here as well. Rheumatoid arthritis and osteoarthritis, the two most common rheumatic diseases, are characterized by stiff, sore, and swollen joints. The latter is considered a wear-and-tear affliction where the cartilage inside one or more joints breaks down. Rheumatoid arthritis is an autoimmune disorder in which membranes lining the joints become inflamed and swollen. Some foods seem to make it worse—an indication that the inflammation may be an allergic response.

Both forms of arthritis, but particularly rheumatoid, may improve after eliminating meats, acids, sugar, caffeine, fried foods, salt, chocolate, and plants of the nightshade family (tomatoes, potatoes, eggplant, and tobacco— another reason to give up smoking).

In a Norwegian study, people with rheumatoid arthritis showed significant improvement after they fasted on vegetable juices for ten days, then eliminated eggs, dairy products, sugar, and citrus fruits for three to five months, finally returning to a diet of dairy products and vegetables.

A group of Harvard researchers has found that chicken collagen, a protein in bones and connective tissue, alleviated symptoms of rheumatoid arthritis by disarming the T cells that attack host tissues.

A diet rich in omega 3 oils helps reduce rheumatoid inflammation. Sources include oily fish such as mackerel and salmon, purslane, soybeans, butternuts, English walnuts, and walnut and canola oils.

Hot baths and hot packs are often recommended for relaxing muscles and easing connective tissue (see page 126, DEALING WITH BACK PAIN). If your joints are red, hot, and swollen—an indication of inflammation—physical therapist Betty Kautzmann recommends icing the area before using heat.

Keep your weight down. The more pounds you are carrying, the more strain you put on your skeleton and the harder it is to get around. Consider reducing if you are overweight to ease the strain on your joints.

The Arthritis Foundation recommends that you get into the habit of exercising at the same time every day. This is best done when you have the most flexibility and energy and your medication, if you take any, is having the most effect.

Swimming and exercising in water are recommended for arthritis sufferers. Water at about eighty-three degrees has been found to soothe pain and make joints more supple.

The Arthritis Foundation recommends range-of-motion and strengthening exercises as well as recreational exercise. Below is a sample of their range of motion exercises:

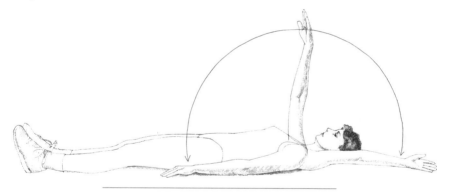

SHOULDER LIE ON YOUR BACK. RAISE ONE ARM OVER YOUR HEAD, KEEPING YOUR ELBOW STRAIGHT. KEEP YOUR ARM CLOSE TO YOUR EAR. RETURN YOUR ARM SLOWLY TO YOUR SIDE. REPEAT WITH YOUR OTHER ARM.

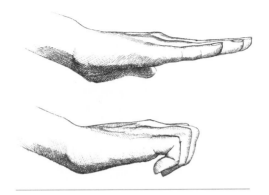

FINGERS OPEN YOUR HAND, KEEPING YOUR FINGERS STRAIGHT.
BEND ALL YOUR FINGER JOINTS EXCEPT YOUR KNUCKLES.
TOUCH THE TOP OF YOUR PALM. OPEN YOUR HAND AND REPEAT.

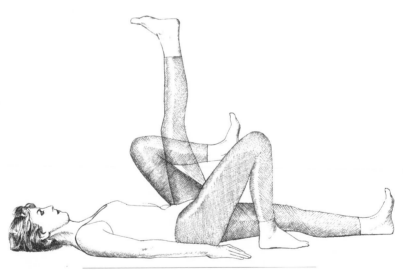

KNEE AND HIP LIE ON YOUR BACK WITH ONE KNEE BENT AND THE OTHER AS STRAIGHT AS POSSIBLE.
BEND THE KNEE OF THE STRAIGHT LEG AND BRING IT TOWARD YOUR CHEST.
PUSH THIS LEG INTO THE AIR AND LOWER IT TO THE FLOOR.
REPEAT WITH THE OTHER LEG.

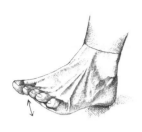 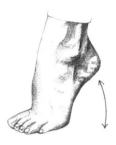

ANKLE WHILE SITTING, KEEP YOUR HEEL ON THE FLOOR AND LIFT YOUR TOES AS HIGH AS POSSIBLE; THEN RETURN YOUR TOES TO THE FLOOR. NEXT, KEEPING YOUR TOES ON THE FLOOR, LIFT YOUR HEELS UP AS HIGH AS POSSIBLE, AND RETURN THEM TO THE FLOOR. REPEAT.

Herbal and Folk Remedies

DR. LUCY SMITH, a naturopathic physician who practices in Seattle, recommends glucosamine sulfate, a natural compound that may normalize cartilage metabolism. In clinical studies, glucosamine sulfate has been shown to regenerate damaged cartilage and exhibit anti-inflammatory activity. Glucosamine sulfate distributors include Bio Therapeutics, P.O. Box 1745, Green Bay, Wisconsin 54305.

THERE IS evidence that aspirin and other nonsteroid painkillers, which many arthritis patients take, may accelerate joint destruction. The herbs devil's-claw and feverfew, both popular folk remedies, have recently been the subjects of clinical studies, proving to be effective in treating pain and inflammation. The suggested daily feverfew dose is $^1/_2$ teaspoon dried herb or three leaves of the fresh herb steeped in boiling water for ten minutes.

DANDELION ROOTS and nettles, both available in health food stores as well as the countryside, are ancient treatments for arthritis, as are herbs containing salicylic acid (the original source of aspirin) such as willow, wintergreen, meadowsweet, and aspen leaves. To take any of these herbs, steep the leaves or boil the roots in boiling water for ten minutes. You can also make a meal of fresh dandelion or nettle greens.

FOR RELIEF of arthritis, Jamaicans swear by a tea made with the island herbs cerasee and fever grass. You can buy these at some herb stores and Korean markets.

SAMUEL CULPEPER, the great English herbalist, held horseradish in high esteem as an arthritis preventative and used it both internally and externally.

VITAMIN E—400 IU a day—may relieve arthritis symptoms in postmenopausal women.

TO HELP flush out uric acid, herbal practitioners often prescribe herbs that have a diuretic effect. Pure water is most frequently recommended. Herbs used for this purpose include goldenrod, a favorite with Native Americans, and black currant juice, used by Europeans to increase the flow of urine. Foods that stimulate the kidneys include watermelon and cucumber (especially the seeds), carrots, watercress, chervil, leeks and onions, asparagus, celery, and parsley.

SAUNAS AND other sweat baths have a universal and ancient reputation for helping remove toxins, including uric acid.

BATHING IN Epsom salts is an old-fashioned palliative for arthritis. Add a cup to your bath. You could also try a handful of chamomile or thyme to ease inflammation. Hot packs of arnica or sweet clover seeds are very soothing. Naturopath Dr. Lucy Smith recommends castor oil packs followed by heat (see pages 107–108 for further instruction).

IN THE Algerian desert, along the beaches of Ecuador, and in other locations where the weather is hot and the sand plentiful, arthritics are buried in hot sand for an hour. Walking in sand is also a good exercise for arthritis.

FOR A penetrating liniment, add one ounce oil of wintergreen to one pint olive or other salad oil. You can replace the wintergreen with other warming and stimulating ingredients such as oil of juniper, angelica, camphor, peppermint, eucalyptus, rosemary, cayenne pepper, or cloves. If you prefer a non-oily mixture, steep a fresh handful or a ground teaspoonful of any of these herbs in a pint of alcohol for a couple of weeks. Before you use it, test yourself for possible allergic reaction by applying the liniment to a small patch of skin. If your skin becomes red and/or irritated, you are sensitive to the ingredients and shouldn't use them.

IN 1994, the *Annals of Internal Medicine* reported that gammalinolenic acid, sold as evening primrose oil in health food stores, is effective at relieving the joint swelling and pain of rheumatoid arthritis.

IN HAITI, compresses are soaked in cider vinegar and applied to cool inflammation and soothe pain.

PERHAPS THE most famous arthritis remedy is Hungary water. Daily rubdowns with it supposedly cured Queen Elizabeth of Hungary from paralysis. The recipe, recorded by Eleanor Sinclair Rhode in *A Garden of Herbs,* calls for one gallon brandy or other spirits, and one handful each of rosemary, myrtle, and lavender, cut in twelve-inch pieces. The brew was steeped for three days and distilled. A modern adaptation would be to steep smaller pieces of the herbs in spirits and place in a sunny window for a couple of weeks.

Back Pain

An overworked, strained, or torn muscle can result in back pain; so can a stretched or torn disk. Although the pain, which can range from a dull ache to a sharp stab, may come on suddenly, the injury is likely to be the result of cumulative stress. If you suffer from repeated or persistent back pain, seek a diagnosis from a licensed health care provider such as a rheumatologist, physiatrist, physical therapist, orthopedist, chiropractor, or osteopath who is trained to identify the many possible causes for back pain. Recent clinical studies suggest that inactivity is not the most effective treatment. The *New England Journal of Medicine* reported that people who resumed their normal activities made the best recovery. Check with your health care provider.

Dealing with back pain

The Physical Medicine and Rehabilitation Center in Englewood, New Jersey, and Betty Kautzmann, the center's Chief Physical Therapist and founder of Englewood Hospital's "Back School," offer these tips:

- To relieve pressure on your disks and surrounding nerves, cushion your face and chest with pillows (a towel roll for your forehead and a pillow under your chest) and lie facedown for ten to twenty minutes every three or four hours.

- Heat, especially wet warmth, can be soothing. Stand in a hot shower, apply a wet compress, or lay a warm wet washcloth over the area for fifteen or twenty minutes. After a while, your skin temperature drops to compensate for the heat, so don't apply heat for longer than twenty minutes. **Warning:** During pregnancy, heat is not a good treatment for back pain because it increases your core temperature and may harm the fetus.

- Walk, swim, or do other moderate exercise as soon as it's comfortable. Avoid sports that require prolonged sitting or repeated bending or twisting such as rowing, bicycling, racket sports, baseball, and the like.

- Prolonged sitting, coughing, sneezing, straining, twisting, bending, bouncing, or heavy lifting can aggravate the problem. Correct your work and recreation posture, and deal promptly with coughs, sneezes, and constipation to allow your back to rest and heal.

- If you must sit when you work, drive, or travel, provide lumbar support with a rolled towel secured with a rubber band or a small pillow placed

at the small of your back. Sit with your back straight, knees higher than your hips, and get up every thirty to forty-five minutes, place your hands on your lower back, and lean back. Repeat ten times.

- To avoid stress on your disks and lower spine, pivot from your feet rather than your waist.

- Balance your weight as much as possible: stand so your weight is distributed equally on both feet; wear a backpack over both shoulders; and use both hands to carry parcels and luggage so the weight is balanced. This is especially important during pregnancy, when hormonal changes make your ligaments stretch and relax, so your body is loose and you may not have as much support as you need.

- To spare your back unnecessary bending and twisting, pack perishable groceries separately so you can unpack and refrigerate them at the same time.

- Sleep on your back with a pillow under your knees or on your side with a pillow between your knees. If you raise one foot before you roll out of bed it places less strain on your back.

- When vacuuming, lead with your feet, not your head. Wrap the hose around your back so you don't put your head in front of your lead foot.

- When ironing, relieve the strain on your back by standing with one foot slightly raised and supported by a telephone book. The lower shelf of a cupboard also works as a footrest.

- Exercise to strengthen your abdominal muscles so they can carry some of the weight. For example, lie on the floor with knees bent, and grasp your opposite leg.

To strengthen abdominals, Suzanne Gosselin, B.S.N., D.C., a Rockport, Massachusetts chiropractor, recommends this sit-back exercise, an easier version of the sit-up:

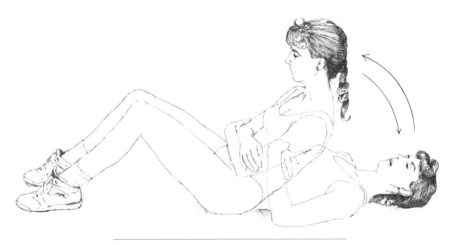

SIT ON THE FLOOR WITH YOUR ARMS FOLDED ACROSS YOUR CHEST, KNEES BENT, AND FEET FLAT ON THE FLOOR. TILT YOUR PELVIS SO THE SMALL OF YOUR BACK FLATTENS SLIGHTLY. HOLD THIS POSITION WHILE ROLLING BACK TO LIE DOWN, TAKING SEVEN SECONDS TO DO SO. USE YOUR ARMS TO HELP YOURSELF SIT UP. REPEAT THE SIT-BACK FIVE TO TEN TIMES TWICE A DAY. DOING A SIT-BACK WITH YOUR ARMS HELD OUT IN FRONT OF YOU IS AN EVEN EASIER VERSION.

Much of our back, neck, and shoulder discomfort comes from what Dr. Gosselin terms "the microtrauma of daily living," tiny insults to the musculoskeletal system that result from misuse and strain.

New York City Alexander Technique instructor Hope Martin states that habits that cause pain, poor posture, and fatigue are established early in life and become reinforced as the years go on. For example, as you read this, are you using muscles that contribute to excessive bodily tension? Can you drop your shoulders and use less muscular effort to hold the book? Can you allow more length through your spine and a fuller, freer breath?

Your head is heavy, Martin reminds us, weighing about fourteen pounds. If it is not poised and balanced on the top of your spinal column, the weight presses down on your neck and compresses your entire spine, interfering with free movement of your arms and legs, contributing to shoulder tension, and diminishing the easy functioning of your organs, breathing mechanism, and voice.

To observe this phenomenon, says Martin, try this simple exercise. Put your fingers lightly in your ears. If they could touch, your fingers would be at the top of your spine. Next, suggests Martin, imagine the muscles that attach to your neck and the base of your skull. When these muscles are contracted, they pull the weight of your head down on your spine. Most of us contract our neck muscles unconsciously without even noticing how it affects us. Shut your eyes and notice how these shortened muscles pull your head down, compressing your spine and affecting your breathing. The weight may pull your shoulders forward as well, notes Martin. Notice how your contracted muscles affect your body and your state of mind.

Back-saving tips by Hope Martin, certified member of the North American Society of Teachers of the Alexander Technique; her practice is in New York City:

- When you sit or stand, allow the tight muscles in your neck to let go so that the crown of your head can float up toward the ceiling. You should feel a sense of maximum ease and poise and opening as your head rests on top of your spinal column so that there's no compression whatever through your spine. Shut your eyes and note the effect of this on your body, your breathing, and your state of mind.

- When you stand, visualize your entire spine from your ears to your tailbone. As you walk, notice what part of your torso initiates the movement. Does your neck jut forward and your chin lead the movement? Or do your shoulders, pelvis, or ribs lead the movement forward?

- When you walk, allow your neck muscles to release so the crown of your head floats up. Let your legs move forward as your spine continues to lengthen in an upward direction. Allow your spine to elongate to its optimum length as your legs take you forward in space.

- Focus on what you are doing rather than the goal or end result. Let the impulse to lengthen come from the thought of releasing tight muscles in your neck, which allow your head to float up, then your spine to lengthen. The operative word here is "allow." You don't want to create more tension by forcefully moving already tight muscles.

Broken Bones

Although a broken bone is a medical problem where you should certainly seek professional help, there are some at-home strategies that may help you recover more quickly. As with any other part of your body, if your bones are strong and healthy before injury, they will heal more readily. Taking in at least 1,000 milligrams of calcium a day, avoiding caffeine, alcohol, tobacco, and other substances that promote bone loss, and getting plenty of weight-bearing exercise are health habits that strengthen your skeletal system. (Dairy products, canned sardines and salmon with the bones in, tofu, blackstrap molasses, broccoli, kale, and legumes are rich in calcium.)

Herbal and Folk Remedies

IN SAUDI Arabia, scientists have found that peppergrass, taken orally, helps speed bone healing.

"KNITBONE," ONE of the nicknames for the herb comfrey, indicates a traditional use—as a poultice to ease painful joints and bones. Allantoin, one of its chemical constituents, is a cell-proliferant that helps repair damaged tissue. **Note:** Apply only to unbroken skin and do not use internally.

IN JAMAICAN folk medicine, a broken foot is wrapped in a cloth soaked in a solution of 1/4 cup salt to one pint vinegar. The compress is kept hot from twenty-four to forty-eight hours, until the foot can be flexed and the bones pulled gently into place.

Bursitis

Bursitis is an inflammation of the fluid sac (bursa) that normally minimizes friction between tendons and bone or bone and bone. The shoulder is a typical site, but bursitis can occur at any joint in the body.

Coping with bursitis
Advice from chiropractor Suzanne Gosselin:

- Bursitis is often the result of physical stress to muscles. Muscle tension may compress the joint, which in turn compresses the bursa so it becomes inflamed.

- Restrict excessive activity of the involved area so the joint can rest.

- Apply ice to the joint for about ten minutes once an hour.

- Use a natural anti-inflammatory substance to ease pain. The herbs feverfew, chamomile, and ginger are anti-inflammatory. Infuse a teaspoon of the dried herb (or boil three slices raw gingerroot) in boiling water for ten minutes.

- To prevent further injury, you need to deal with muscle tension. Stretching exercises are very good for this.

The stretching and strengthening exercises below are recommended for shoulder problems by the Physical Medicine and Rehabilitation Center in Englewood, New Jersey:

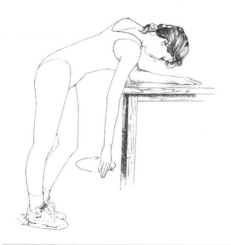

CODMAN'S PENDULUM LEAN FORWARD SO YOUR INJURED ARM HANGS STRAIGHT DOWN IN A RELAXED POSITION. GENTLY SWING YOUR ARM IN CLOCKWISE CIRCLES, THEN IN COUNTERCLOCKWISE CIRCLES.

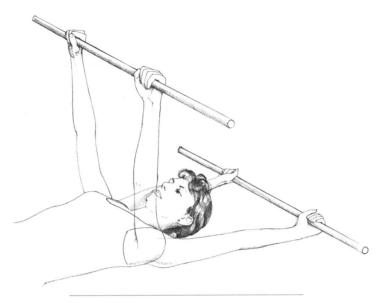

FORWARD ELEVATION LIE FLAT ON YOUR BACK, PALMS UP, GRASPING A BAR WITH BOTH HANDS. RAISE BOTH HANDS OVER YOUR HEAD AS FAR AS POSSIBLE, HOLD FOR FIVE SECONDS, LOWER YOUR ARMS, AND REPEAT.

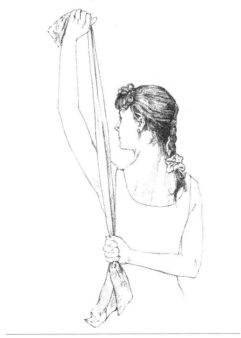

INTERNAL ROTATION GRASP THE END OF A TOWEL OR BAR WITH THE HAND ON YOUR INJURED SIDE. PUT THE UNINVOLVED HAND BEHIND YOUR BACK AT ABOUT WAIST LEVEL AND GRASP THE OTHER END OF THE BAR OR TOWEL WITH IT. PULL AT THE END OF THIS OBJECT WITH THE HAND BEHIND YOU SO THE OTHER ARM IS RAISED AS HIGH AS POSSIBLE. REPEAT.

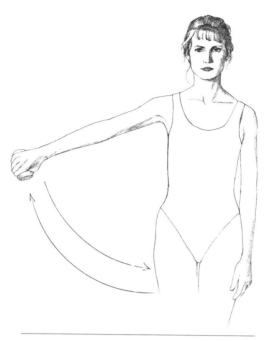

STRENGTHENING STAND WITH YOUR ELBOW STRAIGHT, HOLDING A FIVE-POUND WEIGHT, HAND ROTATED INWARD SO THE BACK OF YOUR HAND FACES FRONT. RAISE YOUR ARM SO IT IS ALMOST LEVEL WITH YOUR SHOULDER (ABOUT SEVENTY DEGREES). HOLD FOR TWO SECONDS, LOWER, REPEAT.

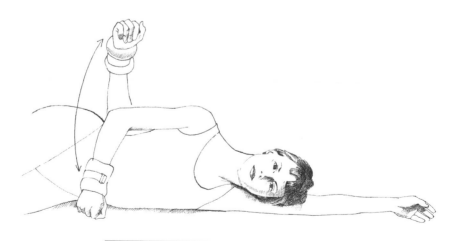

STRENGTHENING LIE ON YOUR UNINVOLVED SIDE, YOUR HEAD ON YOUR UNINVOLVED ARM. WEARING A WRIST-WEIGHT, HOLD YOUR INJURED ARM PARALLEL WITH YOUR BODY, ELBOW BENT AT A NINETY-DEGREE ANGLE, HAND CLOSED IN A FIST, PALM DOWN. RAISE AND ROTATE YOUR FOREARM SO IT IS AT A NINETY-DEGREE ANGLE TO YOUR SIDE AND YOUR PALM IS FACING FORWARD. HOLD FOR TWO SECONDS, LOWER, REPEAT.

Feet

Women's feet, symbolic and real foundations for independence, have traditionally been squashed into high-heeled, pointy-toed pumps, if not actually crippled by immobilizing bindings, as was the custom in some parts of Asia. Now that sneakers are socially acceptable, corns and bunions may become history.

Tight socks can be as confining as tight shoes, and loose socks can bunch up, wrinkle, and raise blisters, so make sure that yours fit properly.

After age forty, check your shoe size every year or so. Our feet spread as we age and the ligaments that hold our bones in place grow less elastic.

Bunions

A painful swelling on the side of the big-toe joint, a bunion forms when the big toe is pulled out of alignment. The cause is overpronation (landing on the outside of your foot). Tight shoes aggravate the problem.

To prevent bunions from forming or recurring, it helps to avoid shoes that narrow at the toe. A corrective device inside your shoe will cushion the swelling and correct pronation.

Herbal and Folk Remedy

A RUSSIAN folk remedy for both bunions and loafer bumps (swellings below the Achilles tendon caused by friction with the back of your shoe) is mashed garlic moistened with kerosene. Cover with plastic or wool overnight.

Corns

These painful swellings with hard cores, often caused by tight footwear, can be smoothed down with a pumice stone, emery board, or sandpaper. Wear moleskin in your shoes to cushion the swellings. Trimming the corn with a razor is best done by your doctor.

Ingrown Toenail

An ingrown toenail occurs when the sides of a toenail (usually on the big toe) grow into the tip of a toe. The resulting injury can be painful and become infected.

To avoid ingrown nails, clip them straight across and avoid tight footwear that can press the edges of your toenails into the surrounding flesh.

If the area is painful, soak your feet in hot water or an Epsom salt solution, and gently insert a piece of cotton under the nail to cushion your skin.

Fibromyalgia

Notoriously underdiagnosed, fibromyalgia, or myofascial pain syndrome, is a muscular condition that resembles arthritis or pinched nerves. The main causes are injury or repeated physical stress. "Trigger points," or tender nodules, develop, causing pain and stiffness. Symptoms include tension headaches, stiff neck, and a sensation of muscular tension, as if the muscles were knotted up. The problem is most common among women of child-bearing age. It is often associated with poor restorative sleep and can be aggravated by cold drafts, humid weather, and emotional stress.

Preventing and relieving fibromyalgia
Advice from physiatrist Howard Liss, M.D., a director of the Physical Medicine and Rehabilitation Center in Englewood, New Jersey; Director of Sports and Musculoskeletal Rehabilitation at Columbia-Presbyterian Medical Center; and Assistant Clinical Professor of Rehabilitation Medicine at Columbia University:

- Poor posture can result in fibromyalgia. Stand or sit with your spine straight, not slumped or swaybacked, and the crown of your head flat (see "Back-saving tips" on page 128 for details).

- Do some form of aerobic exercise for twenty minutes three times a week, reaching a therapeutic heart rate two-thirds of your maximal heart rate (220 plus your age).

- Ice the trigger points (see illustration on page 135), then press your finger hard into these tender points for ten to thirty seconds each, and follow by stretching the involved muscles.

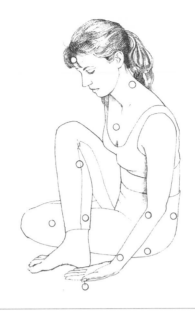

FIBROMYALGIA TRIGGER POINTS

Studies at the Mayo Clinic in Rochester, Minnesota have shown that medical students deprived of stage IV, the deepest stage of sleep, woke with symptoms similar to fibromyalgia. Once stage-IV sleep was restored, their symptoms disappeared.

Muscle Cramps

Muscle fatigue, poor circulation, electrolyte imbalance, or dehydration can cause muscle cramps.

Chiropractor Suzanne Gosselin advises that heavy laxative or diuretic use can deplete our magnesium, so you should be sure to eat plenty of nuts, soybeans, dark leafy greens and other magnesium-rich foods.

Rub the muscle with massage oil or liniment made with arnica.

To restore the electrolyte balance, Dr. Rudolph Weiss, author of *Herbal Medicine,* recommends the following mixture: one teaspoon each peppermint and fennel seed steeped for ten minutes in one liter (one quart plus 3 tablespoons) water, $^1/_2$ teaspoon salt, $^1/_4$ teaspoon bicarbonate of soda, $^1/_4$ teaspoon potassium chloride, two teaspoons glucose.

Neck Pain

Whether temporary or chronic, a pain in the neck is such a common nuisance that it has become a synonym for aggravation. Symptoms can range from fleeting stiffness to crippling muscle spasms. The range of causes can be equally wide—from a cold draft to arthritis, osteoporosis, or whiplash.

Poor posture and tension can aggravate or even cause a stiff neck. Keep your spine straight, the crown of your head flat, and don't slump. See page 128 for details on posture.

Preventing and relieving neck pain
Advice from chiropractor Dr. Suzanne Gosselin:

- A pillow should provide you with support, not just comfort. Mostly it needs to support your neck in a neutral position so it isn't twisted, strained, or bent. In order to do this, your spine should be in a straight line. To find out if you are sleeping correctly (i.e., without straining your neck), lie in your favorite sleep position and have someone come in and look at you. If you are lying on your back in a well-supported position, they should see your chin pointing toward your feet, your forehead parallel with the ceiling, and your ears in line with your shoulders. If you are lying on your side, the bump at the back of your skull should be in a straight line with your backbone, and your ears should be relatively in line with your shoulders.

- A cervical pillow may be helpful, since it is designed to cradle your head correctly and support your neck. Some individuals find that a neck roll—a cloth cylinder filled with foam or buckwheat hulls—can also be effective.

Certain activities that cause you to tilt your head back contribute to neck strain. Don't drive an automobile with your chin up, sit near the front of a church, auditorium, or theater, drink from a can or bottle, read a newspaper unfolded, apply paint or do other work on overhead objects.

When driving, use mirrors as much as possible so you won't have to twist around; when you must turn, keep your chin down and turn with your whole body. Keep your hands low on the steering wheel, adjust the seat forward so you can reach the pedals easily, and be sure the head restraint is level with the back of your head.

If you work at a computer, adjust the terminal so it is at eye level, especially if you wear glasses. (See illustration on page 143.) Use a copy holder that attaches to the side of your computer at eye level.

Don't hold your head against gravity for long periods of time. For example, when you are writing, doing desk work, or sewing, take a break every twenty or thirty minutes and walk around tall. (See page 128 on posture.)

Hold your head straight when talking on the telephone; don't lean toward the receiver or tuck the handset under your chin.

When swimming, stick to the side- or backstroke; the breaststroke and crawl strain your neck.

Rest in bed after an injury to allow the strained muscles to heal. Sleep only on your side or back, and be sure the pillow fills the space between your neck and shoulder.

For the first twenty-four to forty-eight hours after an injury, apply ice, using a cervical pack or a paper cup, for fifteen minutes or less, once an hour. Later you can use moist heat at hourly intervals for no longer than twenty minutes. To apply moist heat, use hot compresses or stand in a hot shower with a heavy towel draped around your neck and shoulders.

If you must sit for long periods of time, take frequent exercise breaks.
A few are described and illustrated below:

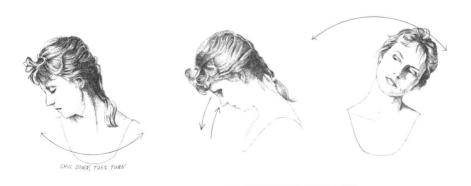

CHIN DOWN, THEN TURN

ROTATE YOUR HEAD FORWARD AND FROM SIDE TO SIDE SEVERAL TIMES TO LOOSEN NECK MUSCLES.

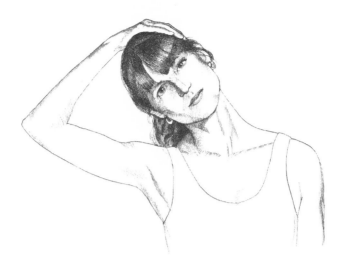

TO STRETCH YOUR NECK MUSCLES, LET YOUR ARM THAT IS ON THE SAME SIDE AS THE SORE NECK MUSCLE HANG LOOSE. RAISE THE OPPOSITE ARM, GRASP YOUR HEAD, AND PULL GENTLY. REPEAT FIVE TIMES.

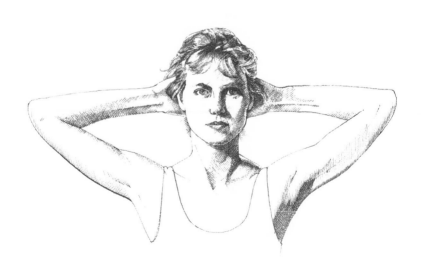

TO STRENGTHEN YOUR NECK MUSCLES, FOLD YOUR HANDS BEHIND YOUR HEAD AND PUSH YOUR HEAD AGAINST YOUR RESISTING HANDS. REPEAT FIVE TIMES.

Osteoporosis

Osteoporosis is characterized by increasingly porous and brittle bones that break easily, even during normal everyday activities such as lifting, bending, coughing or sneezing. Wrist and hip fractures and compression fractures of the spine are the most common. Although some men do have osteoporosis in later years, it is mainly a disease of postmenopausal women, linked with the decline in estrogen. Hormone replacement therapy is usually recommended for women who have a family history of the disease.

If you chose not to undertake hormone replacement therapy, natural progesterone, applied externally, may actually help prevent or alleviate osteoporosis, according to Dr. John Lee, its leading proselytizer. The cream is available from Professional and Technical Services, Inc., 3331 N.E. Sandy Boulevard, Portland, Oregon 97232-1926. 1-(800) 648-8211.

Dr. Evelyn P. W. Whittock, author of *The Calcium Plus Workbook*, notes that a number of substances inhibit calcium absorption or promote its loss. These include cortisone and other steroids, nonsteroid anti-inflammatory drugs (NSAIDS), certain blood pressure medications and diuretics, and antacids containing aluminum. She points out that severely anorexic women who stop menstruating may suffer bone loss because they are not manufacturing enough estrogen. She adds that studies show breast-feeding, if it is accompanied by good nutrition, seems to promote bone-building.

Preventing osteoporosis
Advice from Lisa Long, M.P.T., Assistant Chief Physical Therapist at the Physical Medicine and Rehabilitation Center in Englewood, New Jersey:

- A silent disease until a bone breaks, osteoporosis is most common in small-boned, postmenopausal women, particularly those of Caucasian or Asian descent.

- To prevent and/or minimize osteoporosis, it is important to have good nutritional and exercise habits throughout life. Strong healthy bones are built in childhood and adolescence, and peak bone mass is achieved between the ages of thirty and thirty–five The greatest bone density loss occurs in the first year or two after menstruation ceases. If you have a higher bone density before menopause and maintain good nutritional, postural, and exercise habits during and after, you will be better able to resist the deleterious effects of osteoporosis, such as fractures and postural changes.

- People with a high lifetime calcium intake do have stronger bones. At least 1,000 milligrams a day, equivalent to about a quart of milk, and 1,500 milligrams a day during pregnancy, lactation, and during and after menopause are the minimum requirements. It is equally important to have adequate amounts of magnesium in your diet in order for calcium to be better absorbed. A two to one ratio of calcium to magnesium is suggested.

- Avoid alcohol, caffeine, and tobacco, which can leach calcium from your bones and put you at higher risk for the disease.

Many women are concerned about the current practice of adding growth hormones and antibiotics to milk. Organic milk sold in health food stores is free of hormones and additives, and some dairies that sell to supermarkets also supply milk that is hormone- and additive-free. That information is usually displayed on the milk container or posted near the dairy case.

Other calcium sources include sardines with bones (372 milligrams calcium per serving, while an eight-ounce glass of skim milk is 302 milligrams), salmon with bones, tofu, blackstrap molasses, kale, and dried beans. Leafy green vegetables such as spinach and beet and turnip greens, although excellent calcium sources, contain oxalic acid, which prevents your digestive system from absorbing the calcium. If you eat these greens, which are otherwise packed with nutrients, be sure to take in extra calcium with your meal.

Although calcium is better absorbed from foods, you can take supplements, but make sure they will dissolve properly in your intestines. Test your tablets by placing one in vinegar for about half an hour. If the tablet breaks up, it will dissolve in your stomach (provided that your stomach is producing an adequate amount of hydrochloric acid).

In several American and British studies, bone loss has been associated with magnesium deficiency. A daily supplement of 600 milligrams a day may actually increase bone density. Chiropractor Dr. Suzanne Gosselin observes that loading up on calcium leaches out magnesium. If you do take calcium supplements, look for ones that contain both vitamin D and magnesium.

Vitamin D is a potent accompaniment to calcium, as it helps absorption and maintains the calcium–phosphorus balance.

The link between weight-bearing exercise and bone density has been well established. Walking, jogging, and weightlifting are among the best for stimulating your long bones to produce new cells. Weightlifting stabilizes your joints, decreases pain, and increases mobility, says Dr. Maria A. Fiatrone, chief of the physiology lab at the USDA Human Nutrition Center on Aging at Tufts University.

You can also strengthen your upper body by doing wall pushups. To do these, brace yourself against a wall with your hands, then fall toward the wall and push yourself back with your hands. To increase bone density in your forearms, squeeze a tennis ball for thirty seconds.

Too much exercise may be as bad as too little, however, according to a Stanford University study which found that women in their late fifties who exercised more than five hours a week had a bone density as low as that of nonexercising women in their late sixties.

Weightlifting tips from Carole Taylor Schanley, Fitness Instructor and Director of Move It to Music in Manchester by the Sea, Massachusetts:

- Women tend to fear weight training, thinking it will result in huge muscles. However, female hormones don't encourage muscular overdevelopment. Working up to five or ten pound weights is an adequate goal for most women and unlikely to result in large muscles.

- In addition to increasing bone density, weightlifting, like other forms of exercise, can strengthen your immune system and contribute to good mental health. Weight and resistance training strengthens your quadriceps muscles, which in turn will protect your knees—a body area that is prone to sports injuries. Strengthening your abdominals by doing crunches (partial sit-ups) also acts as a protective device for your back muscles. Like most regular exercise, weight training also raises your metabolism, so you use up more calories even when you are not exercising. Remember: it takes more calories to sustain muscle mass than fat.

- The best way to begin weight training is to take a class. Self-taught weightlifters can easily injure themselves, and the sort of injury you get from lifting weights incorrectly may take a long time to heal. For at-home sessions between classes, work along with a videotape that demonstrates proper technique.

- To avoid strain, don't work the same muscles hard two days in a row. The most effective schedule for training would be alternate days two or three times a week for twenty to thirty minutes. Alternating or combining weightlifting with Yoga or stretching exercises helps you develop and maintain flexibility.

- With aerobic exercise such as running, you know when you need to take a breath, so you naturally breathe correctly then. In my classes, however, I often have to remind participants to breathe steadily when they are working hard. Never hold your breath.

• You need oxygen for optimum performance. Time your breathing so you exhale when you are exerting the most effort, such as when you are lifting hand weights. Inhale as you lower the weights.

Repetitive Stress Injury

In terms of dollars spent on medical care, repetitive stress injuries are surpassing low-back injuries, notes chiropractor Suzanne Gosselin. A great many musculoskeletal disorders, she says, are caused by "the microtrauma of daily living." Think of repetitive actions as drops that fill up a teacup, says Dr. Gosselin. When the accumulated drops fill the cup to overflowing, you start having repetitive stress symptoms. Some examples include sports injuries such as tennis elbow or shin splints. More common are the headaches, neck strains, or disorders of the back, shoulders, or legs caused by the work environment.

Preventing and relieving repetitive stress injury
Advice from chiropractor Dr. Suzanne Gosselin:

• Women are often afflicted by repetitive stress injuries, in part because hormones affect biochemistry. For example, during premenstrual syndrome, pregnancy, and menopause, your tissues lose essential nutrients, including vitamin B6 and magnesium, both essential to proper functioning of the nervous and musculoskeletal systems. Heavy use of alcohol, caffeine, and diuretics also deplete our store of B6. Swelling of the soft tissues can result. Many B vitamins don't work in isolation, so take a B complex vitamin or—better—eat foods rich in the vitamin B complex. Meats, especially liver, are good sources of most B vitamins, so

are wheat germ, soybeans, and brewer's yeast.

• Women are advised to load up on calcium, but too much of it plays havoc with your magnesium level. If your health care provider thinks it would be beneficial for you to take a calcium supplement, buy a good brand—one that includes magnesium—for you usually get what you pay for.

• A major culprit in repetitive stress injuries is the work stations we are expected to use. Even a perfect one creates stress and injuries because it is never designed for one individual's needs. A comfortable work station can enable you to work for longer periods without fatigue or strain. Set up your desk, chair, and computer so you are looking straight ahead, ears over your shoulders. Orient the computer screen to eye level, with a copy holder attached to the side so your copy is also at eye level. The keyboard should be directly in front of you.

- Sometimes it is easier to adapt a chair to your anatomy than a desk. The seat and back of a good steno chair can be raised and lowered. Your feet should be supported by a movable footrest or a small stool—dangling feet can impede blood flow.

- Your weight should be balanced on both feet, with a ninety-degree angle at your knees and hips. Try not to lean forward, but align your shoulders over your hips. Avoid reaching up or forward with your arms. Ideally, your arms should be at your sides, shoulders relaxed, at a ninety-degree angle at your elbows. Keep your elbows below your shoulders, wrists in neutral position, not flexed. (See illustration below.)

- Every half hour, change your body tension for maybe thirty seconds by reaching up, leaning back, stretching, taking a deep breath. In this way you offset being pulled forward and in by opening up and releasing muscle tension. (See illustration on page 144.)

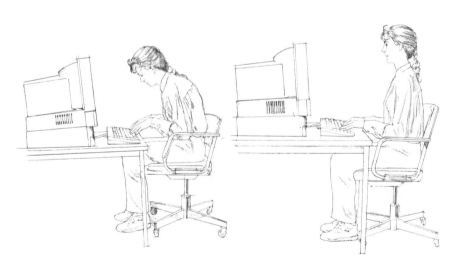

SLUMPED POSTURE AND FLEXED WRISTS
CAUSE STRAIN

CORRECT POSTURE WITH BACK STRAIGHT,
WRISTS SUPPORTED

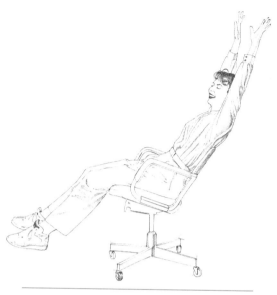

TAKE A THIRTY SECOND BREAK EVERY HALF HOUR: LEAN BACK, STRETCH, TAKE A DEEP BREATH.

Carpal Tunnel Syndrome

Because so many women work at computers, carpal tunnel syndrome (CTS) is one of the most common repetitive stress injuries. The women most likely to be affected are those between the ages of forty and sixty who type, operate machinery, or perform other repetitive work.

The tendons of ten muscles pass through your carpal tunnel, a narrow channel formed by your wrist bones and ligaments. Because this tunnel is so crowded, friction caused by repetitive motion can irritate your tendons, causing swelling and inflammation, and compressing the nerve that supplies sensation to your thumb and first three fingers. This nerve sends out tingling, numbness, and burning or shooting pain that usually gets worse at night. Rheumatoid arthritis, pregnancy, or diabetes may be contributing factors. It helps to adjust your posture and seating to help minimize wrist flex, and use tools that are easy to grasp without bending your wrists.

Initial treatment should be rest, ice, compression, and elevation (RICE), as in sports injuries. (See page 147.)

To reduce inflammation and pain, drink chamomile, ginger, or feverfew tea.

In a University of Texas study, riboflavin and vitamin B6 relieved symptoms. Allan L. Bernstein, Chief of Neurology at Kaiser Hospital, recommends 150 milligrams of B6 daily. An overdose can be toxic to your nervous system. Do not take if you are pregnant, and when discontinuing use, don't stop abruptly. (To avoid these problems, take a B complex vitamin or food supplement such as brewer's yeast.)

Avoiding or relieving carpal tunnel syndrome—
Advice from Massachusetts chiropractor Suzanne Gosselin:

- A soft-tissue injury that doesn't show up on an X ray, this stress injury often goes undiagnosed until it is advanced.

- If you work at a computer, place the keyboard directly in front of you and put a wrist pad at the base of the keyboard to keep your wrist in a neutral (not flexed) position.

- Take a thirty-second break every half hour and shake your hands. This is a natural wrist relaxer.

- The forearm muscles that work your wrists need to be stretched every half hour or so. To do this, extend one arm from the shoulder straight out in front of you, locking the elbow. With the other hand, passively flex the wrist of your outstretched arm to point the fingers to the ceiling. Hold for a count of five to ten seconds,

then flex your wrist in the other direction so your fingers are pointing toward the floor. Again, hold for five to ten seconds. Repeat on the other side.

- There are many muscles in your hands and fingers, and they respond to overworking and overload. Heat does relax your muscles, so immersing your hands in hot water may relieve stiffness. If you have been pushing yourself and there is swelling, use ice instead of heat. (The latter aggravates inflammation.)

- To stretch your hands, hold them at a ninety-degree angle to your forearm and form a tepee with your fingers. Push the heel of your hands together, then your fingertips and fingers. Bend your fingers back.

Shoulder Discomfort

Most shoulder problems result from wear and tear on the rotator cuff, a group of four muscle/tendon units that are responsible for certain motions of the shoulder joint. Because the flexibility of your shoulder allows for a wide range of activities, and circulation to this area is limited, you are likely to have rotator cuff problems as you get older, especially if you don't warm up and stretch before you exercise. See pages 146 to 148 in the SPORTS IN-JURIES section for more information.

The Physical Medicine and Rehabilitation Center in Englewood, New Jersey, advises resting the joint by avoiding or curtailing upward and outward movements of your arm. To keep the joint mobile, it recommends the range-of-motion exercises described on pages 121–123. When the pain subsides, it's important that you rehabilitate injured tendons with exercise.

Shoulder pain has many causes. To avoid further damage to the rotator cuff, if pain persists or recurs, you should see a licensed health professional.

Sports Injuries

Exercise is a great way to keep fit and avoid—or at least postpone—a variety of chronic ailments. More women in these health-conscious times are enjoying the benefits. There is always a risk of sudden injury—strains, sprains, broken bones, and so on. Other injuries, such as tennis elbow or runner's knee, are the result of cumulative stress. As we get older, some wear and tear is inevitable, but the stress can also be related to problems with anatomy or posture, or improper playing style or equipment. It's a good idea to get advice about equipment and how to use it safely from a coach, trainer, or other expert.

Vitamin E may help protect your muscles. Physically active people may need more vitamin E to protect against possible muscle damage by free radicals produced by increased oxygen consumption, says Jeffrey Blumberg, F.A.C.N., at Tufts University Research Center on Aging.

Once-a-month skiers and tennis players and weekend athletes are risking injury, warns fitness instructor Carole Taylor Schanley. You need to condition yourself with regular exercise, and you should warm up before and cool down after working out. Preparing to exercise, says Schanley, is like fueling and warming up a car. To raise your metabolism, eat a banana, half a bagel, or some other carbohydrate an hour or so before you exercise.

Moving your legs and arms, as in marching in place, followed by light stretching, is a good pre-exercise warmup, Schanley continues. Never stretch cold muscles, she warns. Do aerobics before you stretch so you won't have sore muscles. Walk around a bit first to get your circulation going.

After a preliminary warmup, Schanley recommends a ten-minute pre-exercise warmup that includes a couple of minutes of stretching followed by three minutes of aerobics, then another five minutes of stretching.

After an aerobic or strength-training session, your muscles feel contracted. You need to return them to a flexible position by cooling down properly. Schanley offers these tips for cooling down:

As your heartbeat quickens, your body calls for more oxygen. If you stop exercising suddenly, the blood pools in your lower body and doesn't have a chance to continue fully traversing your circulatory system. You may feel light-headed. You need to get your pulse rate down. Don't cut off your oxygen too soon. If you end your workout with high-endurance exercise, you want to hit your peak and slow down, stop, and stretch. Exercise at a slower pace for five to ten minutes, then cool down by walking before you stretch.

The RICE Treatment for Sports Injuries

Some inflammation is beneficial in protecting and repairing damaged tissue, but it should be controlled to avoid scarring and reduce swelling and pain. Standard treatment for the first forty-eight to seventy-two hours after a sports injury is RICE:

1. **Rest** the injured part, and don't resume the sport or work activity until you can do so without pain. (Exercising other parts of the body is recommended.)

2. **Ice** the area with a chemical cold bag, cold compresses, or crushed ice wrapped in a towel. Betty Kautzmann recommends substituting a big bag of frozen peas and carrots if you don't have ice, or you can use a mixture of two-thirds crushed ice, one-third alcohol. The ice treatment can be done repeatedly, but only at hourly intervals and for no longer than fifteen minutes at a time. When a muscle is pulled or torn, the American Medical Association advises ice every four hours for the first two to four days.

3. **Compress** the swelling by wrapping it firmly but comfortably in an Ace bandage.

4. **Elevate** the injured part as much as possible to drain fluid from the site.

After the first forty-eight to seventy-two hours, Kautzmann advises either heat or ice, whichever feels more comfortable. For some reason, she says, people who like warm weather respond better to cold, and vice versa. Heat increases blood flow, cold constricts it, but as the tissue warms, heat and ice both numb the injury, so painkillers are often not needed.

If in doubt whether to use heat or cold, chiropractor Dr. Suzanne Gosselin advises ice (unless you have diabetes or circulatory problems). Heat, she says, makes inflammation worse. If there is inflammation in the joint, the area will be swollen; cold acts as an anti-inflammatory. However, chronic or repetitive stress injuries usually respond better to heat, because the aggravated tissues are muscles. Soak in a hot bath or apply a heating pad.

After three to six weeks, when you resume exercise, the AMA recommends ice to reduce swelling and heat to relax muscles, increase circulation, and promote healing. Heat may increase swelling, however, so make sure the area is not swollen before you apply the heating pad or hot water bottle.

Herbal and Folk Remedies

DR. MICHAEL Jacobs, a naturopath in Portland, Oregon, prescribes herbal sedatives and antispasmodics such as lady's slipper, skullcap, and valerian to relax tense muscles, relieve muscle cramps, and promote sleep.

ARNICA, USED in European folk and homeopathic medicine, is very soothing to strained, sprained, and sore muscles and tendons. Health food stores sell it in either an oil or an alcohol base.

Achilles Tendinitis

A gradual inflammation of the Achilles tendon area, this form of tendinitis is the result of repeated tiny tears, often caused by improper shoes, overpronation, running downhill, or running on the ball of your foot. It can also be caused by a shortened tendon that results from habitually wearing high-heeled shoes. The condition is usually more painful just after you get out of bed in the morning or when you begin to run.

Stop running until the injury heals.

Massage the tendon with ice three or four times a day for three to five days, or until symptoms ease.

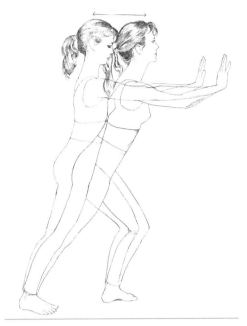

LEAN FORWARD, RESTING YOUR ARMS AGAINST A WALL, WITH YOUR INJURED HEEL ON THE FLOOR AND THE UNINVOLVED LEG BENT AND THRUST FORWARD.

Gently stretch the Achilles tendon and strengthen your back leg muscles with exercises such as the one illustrated above. Another stretching exercise is to sit and raise your toes upward as far as you can, relax, and repeat several times. After a few days, attach a weight to the ball of your foot or instep and repeat the exercise. To stretch your back leg muscles, lie on your back on a table with your foot projecting over the edge. Lift your big toe and rotate the instep side of your foot upward, hold for a few seconds, release, and repeat several times.

Wear a flexible running shoe and use a heel cup or rubber heel wedge in all your footwear. These are soft, flexible devices that fit in the back of your shoe. They help to absorb the shock of walking and running so the tendon is protected from further damage and allowed to heal.

Hamstring Injury

Pain or tenderness in the hamstrings when you bend or sit may be an indication that these large muscles on the back of your thighs are strained or torn. The main cause of this injury is failing to warm up before running. To avoid hamstring injury, stretch as shown in illustration above for ten minutes or so before running or other vigorous exercise.

Ice the area for thirty-six hours. When inflammation has subsided, sit in a warm whirlpool bath. Once the pain has decreased, do gentle stretching exercises such as touching your toes. Avoid running, cycling, rowing, or prolonged driving.

Pain Management

Some tips on pain management from physiatrist Dr. Howard Liss:

- People who do aerobics experience less pain because they produce endorphins (natural painkillers).

- It is important to locate the source of chronic pain. If you know you have an arthritic knee, for example, you can avoid or at least reduce post-exercise discomfort by taking two or three aspirin the day before you plan to exercise to build the anti-inflammatory level in your blood. Be cautious with these drugs if you have asthma, significant hypertension, or kidney disease; do not take them if you have ulcers, gastritis, esophagitis, or esophageal reflex.

Author's Note: To avoid aspirin or other nonsteroidal anti-inflammatory drugs (NSAID) side effects, drink tea made with anti-inflammatory herbs instead. The best ones for this purpose are feverfew, chamomile, and ginger.

Massachusetts chiropractor Suzanne Gosselin recommends ice for a new pain. There is less damage from cold than from heat, she says, because the latter makes inflammation worse. If you have diabetes or circulatory problems, however, you should check with your health care provider.

For chronic injuries, including those caused by repetitive stress, Gosselin advises heat. The aggravated tissues are muscle, she says. Heat soothes pain by relaxing the muscles.

Runner's Knee

The most common running injury is runner's knee, a pain in the knee-cap often caused by pronation, or bearing excessive weight on the inside of your foot. Pronation results from a muscle imbalance or a fault in the structure of your lower extremity bones. It may be corrected by wearing inserts in your walking and exercise shoes. Consult a knowledgeable health practitioner for advice on this orthotic device.

- To improve kneecap tracking, exercise to strengthen the quadriceps, the big muscle at the front of your thigh.
- Chiropractors and osteopaths are trained to evaluate postural problems and joint dysfunctions that may lead to knee and joint problems. You may want to consult one.
- To avoid further injury, stop running. Bike, row, or swim instead. For the first two weeks after the injury, alternate walking and running. By the fourth week you should be able to return to your original running level.

Shin Splints

Shin splints are a form of tendinitis that results in pain along your shin or tibia, the large bone that runs from knee to ankle at the front of your leg. Improper shoes, running on hard or banked surfaces, pronating, and sometimes aerobics can pull at your shins. Continued running may cause stress fractures (hairline cracks) along this bone.

Use ice for three to five days, then alternate with applications of heat and cold. You can engage in light exercise, but wrap your leg in an Ace bandage to provide comfort and support.

When the symptoms disappear, wear an insert prescribed by your health care provider to correct pronation in all your footwear.

Sprains

This common injury is often a tear in the ligament that connects bone to bone. Treat inflammation, swelling, and pain with rest, ice, compression, and elevation, as described on page 147.

Compress the swelling with an Ace bandage. A tight bandage may interfere with circulation, so check with your health care provider if you have diabetes or vascular disease.

After the first two or three days you can start stretching, then, if you feel no pain, do strengthening exercises. If the injury is mild, you can begin stretching and strengthening exercises right away.

For more details, see SPRAINS, page 231 in Chapter Ten, "Emergencies."

Tennis Elbow

The official name is lateral epicondylitis, after the bony ridge (epicondyle) on the outer (lateral) portion of your elbow, where most of your forearm extensor muscles originate. Repetitive activities such as tennis, pitching a softball or baseball, housework, physical labor, and carrying heavy objects result in numerous microtears of these muscles. The epicondyle becomes inflamed, muscle fiber is replaced by scar tissue, and movement gradually becomes stiff and uncomfortable.

To ease discomfort, rest, ice the inflamed area in a circular motion, compress and elevate the injury, as described on page 147. Physical therapist Betty Kautzmann recommends freezing water in a styrofoam cup, then gradually peeling the cup from the ice. The remaining area of styrofoam insulates your hand from the cold.

Wear a tennis elbow splint, wrapped firmly 2 inches below the epicondyle when you use your elbow. Do not wear the splint when you stretch, sleep, or rest your elbow.

As soon as you can tolerate it, stretch the muscles involved with wrist and finger motion.

Below are sample exercises from the Physical Medicine and Rehabilitation Center in Englewood, New Jersey:

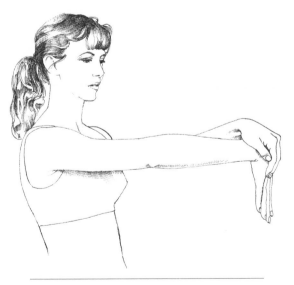

STRETCH EXTEND YOUR INJURED ARM, PALM DOWN, AND WITH THE OTHER HAND GRASP THE BACK OF YOUR EXTENDED HAND AND PUSH YOUR WRIST DOWN AS FAR AS POSSIBLE. HOLD FOR A COUNT OF FIVE. REPEAT TEN TIMES.

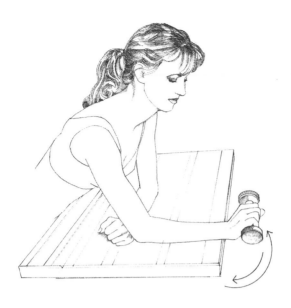

WRIST EXTENSION When the muscle heals, lay your forearm on a table or other flat surface with your hand extending over the edge, grasping a weight. Lower your hand as far as you can, then bring your wrist up. Repeat ten times.

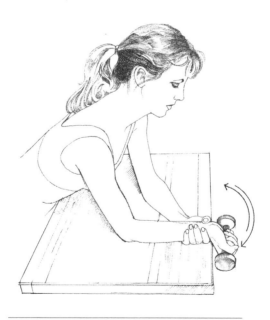

WRIST FLEXION To strengthen and restore wrist flex, follow the directions above with the palm of your hand face up.

To prevent recurrence, you may need to correct your backhand technique, use a dampening device in your racket to absorb shock, or change the size of your racket grip.

Tennis Leg

Advice from physiatrist Dr. Howard Liss:

Associated with racket sports, tennis leg is a tear in your inner calf muscle caused by a contraction of the muscle in the stretch position as you step forward. It is often the result of repeated tiny injuries, but the onset is sudden, and accompanied by a popping sound. The muscle is so tender it cannot be stretched sufficiently to put your heel down. Bruises below the painful area may appear three days after the injury. (**Warning:** If the onset is not sudden and you feel pain not in your inner calf muscle below the midpoint of the leg, but in the middle of your leg, and/or if your ankle is swollen, see a doctor immediately—it could be phlebitis, a serious vascular problem.)

- To reduce inflammation and relieve pain, ice your calf muscle repeatedly at ten-minute intervals and take ibuprofen three times a day—600 milligrams if you weigh under 150 pounds, 800 milligrams if you weigh more.

- Wear a heel lift in your sneakers for the next six weeks, and use a cane or crutches if you still experience sharp pain.

- To gently stretch your calf muscle, lie on the floor with your legs straight. Put a towel under the foot of your injured leg and pull gently, exerting pressure against your foot. Push against the towel with your foot so your calf muscle flexes.

- When healing has progressed to where you can straighten your knee and touch the ground with your injured heel, you can begin stretching exercises to recover your range of motion. Put the injured heel down, straighten that knee, and bend the opposite one. Lean forward, arms bent, forearms and palms flat against a wall. Don't lunge or bounce, but stretch in a sustained position. See illustration on page 149.

- While recovering, you can engage in any sport that does not strain your injured calf muscle, such as biking, swimming, or working out with any upper-body machine.

- When you can stretch both legs symmetrically, you can gradually return to your sport, preferably under the guidance of a physical therapist or physician.

7

The Nervous System:

From Anxiety to Pain

i f the chemicals that are running our body and our brain are the same chemicals that are involved in emotion, we'd better seriously entertain theories about the role of emotions and emotional suppression in disease. We'd better pay more attention to emotions with respect to health.

—Candace Pert, Ph.D., former chief of the section on brain chemistry at the National Institutes of Health, quoted in Bill Moyers, *Healing and the Mind*.

Elsewhere in this book you have read about how stress exacerbates, even triggers disorders in all parts of the body; there is evidence that it can suppress immunity. In this chapter you will read how good nutrition, exercise, and massage can reduce stress, anxiety, depression, and physical pain. The nervous system is the only one where the cells, once they are dead or damaged, do not regenerate. For this reason, long-term alcohol or drug abuse, which destroys brain cells, can cause permanent injury.

Anxiety and Tension

Symptoms of anxiety are familiar to most of us: sweating, sometimes nausea and diarrhea, a racing pulse, perhaps a feeling of dread. Occasions for temporary anxiety are just about endless: starting a new job; getting married or having a baby; taking a test; giving a speech or other public performance; health, money, or family worries.

Anxiety isn't necessarily detrimental—it can be the burr under the saddle that gets you moving. Sometimes all that's needed is to direct those jitters into constructive channels.

An overload of caffeine can produce symptoms of anxiety. Gradually eliminate or at least curtail your caffeine consumption by substituting increasingly larger proportions of decaffeinated tea or coffee. In this way, you may reduce anxiety and avoid caffeine withdrawal symptoms.

Although smokers tend to overindulge when under stress, nicotine is a stimulant, and so likely to increase your tension. Kick the habit and you'll probably find you can take everyday ups and downs more in stride.

Exercise is a great outlet for anxiety because it loosens tense muscles and releases feel-good endorphins. Yoga stretches your muscles and loosens your joints, thereby easing nervous tension. Simple stretching exercises are also helpful.

If your anxiety escalates to a panic attack, advises Carole Taylor Schanley, fitness instructor and director of Move It to Music in Manchester by the Sea, Massachusetts, focus on your breathing. Inhale and exhale twice as slowly as you normally do—it slows you down physically and has a calming effect.

Talking out your problems with a trusted friend or family member can also be an effective way of dealing with temporary anxiety.

Some people do have a lower anxiety threshold than others. However, if you often feel anxious for no apparent reason, or if such feelings persist or interfere with your life, there could be a medical or psychological problem you should discuss with your doctor or a mental health professional.

Herbal and Folk Remedies

YOU PROBABLY have one or more mild sedatives in your kitchen: the phthalide in celery and the serotonin in honey are known to have sedative properties; bread, spaghetti, and other high-carbohydrate foods also have a calming effect. Calcium is another anxiety soother. The recommended daily amount is at least 1,000 milligrams, or the equivalent of a quart of milk.

The Townsend Letter, a periodical directed to naturopathic and homeopathic physicians, recommends 100 milligrams of valerian and 45 milligrams of passionflower (both tranquilizing herbs) taken two or three times a day to decrease anxiety and depression.

OTHER HERB teas that have been sipped for centuries to calm jangled nerves include skullcap, nerveroot (also called lady's slipper), catnip, and hops. Try a teaspoon of one or more of these dried herbs steeped for ten minutes in boiling water.

TO HELP them relax, Africans boil four or five dried orange leaves in a cup of water, add sugar, and drink the hot infusion.

PUERTO RICANS steep three or four fresh leaves of yerbabuena in 1½ cups water for ten minutes or so, add honey, and drink a cup a day. Yerbabuena grows in Puerto Rico and other tropical locales, but you should be able to find it at your local herb or health food supplier.

Depression

At one time or another, we all get the blues. Depression, however, is a pervasive feeling of despondency and worthlessness. It is often accompanied by anxiety. Sleeping or eating too much or too little, inability to concentrate, lack of interest in life or your surroundings, crying spells, and feelings of hopelessness are some of the symptoms of depression, our most common mental illness. Twice as many women as men suffer from it, and women tend to have more adverse reactions to antidepressant medication. If your symptoms last more than a couple of weeks, see your doctor. You could have a hormone or blood sugar imbalance or glandular disease; or you may need counseling and/or medication from a mental health professional.

Sometimes all it takes to banish depression is to concentrate on someone or something outside yourself. The increased self-esteem you derive from accomplishment, or the satisfaction you get from helping someone else can be a sure cure for the blues.

Your blood sugar level affects your moods. A high sugar intake, for example, can give you instant energy. In response to large amounts of sugar, however, the pancreas releases extra insulin, which actually lowers your blood sugar level, resulting in the sugar blues. The best way to stabilize the level of sugar in your blood is to follow a well-balanced, low-sugar diet, with small, frequent meals. Be sure all but your last meal of the day include protein, which slows sugar metabolism.

A woman may feel depressed before her menstrual periods or during menopause because of estrogen fluctuations. Some medical experts believe that natural progesterone may help restore the hormone balance. Try applying $1/8$ to $1/4$ teaspoon progesterone cream to the inside of your arm, chest, or any area where it won't rub off and can be easily absorbed. The cream is sold in health food stores. Regular aerobic exercise releases endorphins—hormones that enhance our sense of well-being.

At menopause there is a drop in blood levels of the mineral magnesium, which is related to lithium, a drug used in treating mood disorders. Be sure your diet includes lots of nuts and whole grains, which are rich in magnesium, and dairy products or soybeans and leafy greens, which are rich in calcium, an important element in maintaining the nervous system.

If you regularly feel depressed during the winter months, you may be suffering from seasonal affective disorder (SAD), a form of depression linked to declining sunlight. For relief, try spending a few hours each day under bright, full-spectrum lighting. Your Yellow Pages or local power company should be able to provide a source for such lights.

The *Journal of the American Medical Association* reports in a 1988 study that some people recovered from depression by altering their sleep patterns. They went to bed earlier and slept less—about five hours a night.

A 1990 Chicago study showed that mild bipolar depression may be relieved by a combination of aerobic exercise, dance therapy, and 500 milligrams of the amino acid L-phenylalanine twice a day along with 50 to 100 milligrams vitamin B6 in the morning.

Researchers at the Touch Institute at the University of Miami Medical School found that a thirty-minute neck and back massage reduced depression in a variety of subjects ranging from adolescent mothers to survivors of Hurricane Andrew. After massage, the subjects were found to have lower levels of the stress-related hormone cortisol and norepinephrine.

Herbal and Folk Remedies

The Townsend Letter reports that the amino acid L-acetylcarnitine, taken 500 milligrams three times a day, has proved helpful in treating depression. The newsletter also reports that a combination of 100 milligrams valerian and 45 milligrams passionflower has been found to decrease anxiety and depression.

SEVERAL STUDIES have been done on the leaves and seeds of ginkgo, an ancient tree species that has been used in Chinese medicine for centuries. Ginkgo has been proven effective in treating depression associated with decreased cerebral blood flow.

Fatigue

The medical causes of fatigue are nearly endless and should be ruled out by a doctor before you try home remedies. Besides physical ailments, depression can also cause fatigue. The most obvious reason for feeling tired is poor-quality or insufficient sleep, a problem in times of stress and during pregnancy and menopause. Burnout and boredom can also leave you feeling as if all your reserves of energy have been depleted.

Poor eating habits and rich, fried, and/or fatty foods can make you feel sluggish. Try a high-protein diet with lots of fresh fruits and vegetables. It is best to get your nutrients from food; if you don't, take supplements.

Instead of making your digestive system work overtime on three hearty meals, eat several small, light ones. This helps your blood sugar, and consequently your energy level, to remain constant.

Coffee, tea, chocolate, tobacco, sugar, and other stimulants can give you a quick lift, but the artificial high can leave you feeling let down afterward. In the short run, most of these don't do you much harm, but in the long run they deplete your energy.

Exercise is energizing. Taking a brisk walk early in the day and after meals will keep your energy up and help ensure a good night's sleep.

Herbal and Folk Remedies

THROUGH THE first half of this century, instead of popping a vitamin pill, people took alteratives when they felt poorly. It was believed that these substances gradually altered the course of disease by stimulating the elimination of tissue wastes. Naturopathy and other forms of alternative medicine still operate on this theory that health is achieved only after toxins are excreted. Herbal alteratives that have traditionally been used include sarsaparilla, Oregon grape, devil's-claw, burdock root, chickweed, dogwood, figwort, blue flag, goldenseal, yellow dock, and spikenard.

TONIC HERBS have been used for centuries to invigorate the glandular system. In China, the herb fo-ti (ho shou wu), available in herb and health food stores, is considered as important to a woman's health and well-being as ginseng is to a man's. It is reputed to energize the nerves, brain cells, and ductless glands and promote longevity. Gotu kola, a botanical relative of fo-ti, is used similarly. Both men and women take it as a brain tonic.

CHINESE LICORICE root is believed to sharpen concentration, improve glandular function, and regulate blood sugar level. Other tonic herbs include gentian, ginseng (Siberian ginseng is more compatible with the female hormonal system), sarsaparilla, willow bark, yarrow, stinging nettle, peach leaves, quassia, European centuary, sage, and chamomile.

Headache

According to the National Headache Society, there are twelve different kinds of headache. Tension headache, caused by head, neck, or shoulder muscle contractions, is probably the most common. The most debilitating are cluster headaches, which involve blinding pain on one side of the head and are mostly suffered by men, and migraines, sometimes known as "sick headache."

The International Headache Registry cites some of the most common causes of headache:

- Overindulgence in food, alcohol or tobacco
- Sleeping too much
- Dieting and fasting
- Sensitivity to red wine, pork, fish, bananas, yogurt, and other foods
- Abrupt temperature changes, such as moving in and out of air conditioning
- Breathing carbon monoxide fumes while driving in heavy traffic
- Noise
- Overdoing physical exercise, especially without warmup
- Sitting or standing in the same position for too long
- High blood pressure
- In rare instances, a brain tumor is also a possible cause of headache

If you have no history of headaches and suddenly get them, if the pain is frequent or severe, or if the headache is accompanied by fever or convulsions or follows a head trauma, see your doctor immediately.

According to the National Headache Society, over-the-counter pain medications such as aspirin can trigger rebound headaches and aggravate the condition. The NHS advises headache sufferers to give up their medication. The symptoms will escalate for the first week, they say, then gradually improve.

Constipation or a sluggish digestive system can cause headache. To improve functioning of your gastrointestinal tract, avoid fats and processed or fried foods, and eat lots of fresh fruit, whole grains, and legumes.

Exercise relieves tension and releases painkiller endorphins; it also improves circulation and digestion—all excellent headache preventatives.

Some headaches result from an abrupt shift in blood flow. This can happen if you get out of bed suddenly in the morning, so get out of bed slowly to allow your blood flow to adjust gradually.

You can get a headache from staying out in the sun too long, especially when the light is intense. A wide-brimmed hat and sunglasses help.

Some studies suggest that stress is a contributing factor in headaches. Recent Australian studies indicate that having a strong support network can provide a buffer for stress and reduce the number of headaches. Try visualization techniques, such as imagining a tranquil scene, to relieve tension or muscle-contraction headaches.

Some people practice deep muscle relaxation to relieve tension headaches: moving from head to toe, tense, then release, specific muscle groups. Moist heat also relaxes muscles and relieves tension. Direct a shower spray to the back of your neck or apply a hot compress or washcloth to the area. The hot water stimulates circulation and decreases muscle waste buildup.

Gentle stretching exercises may relieve headaches caused by tense neck muscles. Yoga, because it stretches neck and spine muscles, is particularly good for tension headaches.

Lying on your back with a rolled towel under your neck can sometimes relieve headache.

Some tension headaches are caused by a chronic contraction of the large muscle that runs from the base of your skull over your shoulders. Massage helps. At times when a masseuse is not available, stroke your right shoulder with your left hand, and vice versa. Work toward your neck, at first lightly, to stimulate circulation, then deeply to break up muscle waste deposits.

For contractions of the large muscle that runs from your temple to your jaw, massage lightly with a natural bristle brush. Using a circular motion, work from the temple along your jaw to your earlobe, then over your ear, to your temple, and down behind your ear to the base of your skull. Do not massage your ear. Repeat the massage four or five times on both sides of your head, beginning each time a little higher on your head.

Poor posture can cause neck strain, resulting in headaches. Don't slouch. Stand and sit so that your spine is straight and the top of your head is level. Don't talk on the phone with the receiver cradled between your neck and shoulder.

Sometimes headache is caused by eyestrain. Be sure you have adequate lighting for reading, writing, sewing, and other close work.

Herbal and Folk Remedies

AFRICANS DRY papaya leaves over a fire, and apply them to their head, which is then wrapped in a handkerchief.

IN THE CARIBBEAN, an aloe vera leaf, split open to expose the gel, is applied to the forehead. Other Caribbean folk remedies include rubbing the head with beer or rum and applying a cold cloth to the forehead. The cold pack works by constricting the engorged blood vessels. A Mexican remedy works on a similar principle: drink very cold water.

Migraine

This intense headache is accompanied by extreme sensitivity to light and noise and preceded by an aura, or blurred vision. Often triggered by stress, migraine is sometimes a response to certain foods such as red wine, chocolate, beef extracts, yeast, cheese, and other fatty dairy items. Blood platelets clump together, releasing serotonin and prostaglandin, which cause the muscles to contract, restricting blood flow and causing intense pain. The traditional treatment is for the migraine sufferer to lie in a dark room and wait until it passes.

Learning to manage stress and avoiding offending foods can help prevent an attack.

Herbal and Folk Remedies

THE HERB feverfew was the eighteenth century's version of aspirin. At London's Chelsea College and the London Migraine Clinic, patients treated with feverfew built resistance to attacks and experienced symptomatic relief. The daily dose is three fresh leaves or a teaspoon of the dried herb infused in a pint of boiling water. The herb can produce an allergic reaction, so start slowly, using about $1/4$ teaspoon of the leaves, and work up to the full amount.

Insomnia

Although eight hours sleep a night is considered standard, individual sleep requirements vary. Some people are fine with five or six hours; others need nine or ten. Many smokers find that they need less sleep after they quit. According to the National Sleep Foundation, it's a myth that as we get older, we need less sleep, but the possibility of a sleep disorder does increase with the passage of time. Older people sleep less at a single stretch than they did when younger, and they get less of the deeper phases of sleep. After the age of sixty-five, the average person wakes for a few seconds as often as 150 times a night.

Sleep researchers have found that natural human sleep patterns are similar to those of some animals. In summer, we tend to sleep less, but we are more likely to sleep through the night. In winter, a natural, though impractical, pattern would be about fourteen hours' sleep interrupted by periods of quiet wakefulness.

Most people experience an occasional day or even week or two of insomnia. If your bouts of sleeplessness are recurrent or last longer than a couple of weeks, it's a good idea to consult a health care professional. Lack of sleep interferes with memory, decreases immunity, and affects your efficiency and sense of well-being.

Battling insomnia
Tips from the National Sleep Foundation:

- Give yourself an hour or so to wind down before bedtime. Be sure your bedroom is dark, quiet, and comfortable, and use it only for sleeping so you'll associate it with rest. Go to bed only when you are sleepy; don't lie in bed when you can't sleep.

- Get up at approximately the same time every day no matter when you went to sleep.

- Keep a sleep log for a few weeks to help you identify and correct behaviors that disrupt your sleep.

Record when you wake up, go to bed, drink caffeinated beverages, exercise, or engage in other suspect behavior.

- Sleeping pills have a role in the treatment of insomnia, but only for transient and short-term situations. If you are a chronic insomniac, you should not depend on sleeping pills to get a good night's sleep. You can become addicted to these drugs, and after your body adapts to their effect, you may need progressively higher doses in order to get to sleep.

Watch your caffeine intake. The drug is metabolized so slowly that half the dose is still circulating through your bloodstream six hours after it is consumed. This means that two cups of coffee at 6 P.M. can have you still awake at midnight.

Alcohol is a stimulant as well as a depressant. Although a nightcap can relax you for sleep, alcohol abuse can cause insomnia and deprive you of the rapid-eye-movement (REM) stage of sleep that helps you maintain emotional stability.

Exercising early in the day helps you get rid of excess energy and relax. Yoga and swimming are particularly good for this. Relaxation exercises help prepare you for sleep, but intense activity close to bedtime will keep you revved up for hours.

Even on weekends, keep to a regular schedule for retiring and rising to train your biological clock. Trying to "catch up" on sleep by getting up later on weekends will make it that much harder to sleep and wake on your weekday schedule. Try going to bed earlier on weekends instead.

Researchers have found that a midday nap actually helps ensure a sound night's sleep. However, this, too, must be done on a regular schedule: erratic napping results in fragmented nighttime sleep.

A high-protein meal is a great way to keep your energy level up, but you don't want that at bedtime. Save the protein for breakfast and lunch; at night, dine on complex carbohydrates (fruits, vegetables, and grain). Digesting a heavy evening meal can keep you awake well into the night. On the other hand, don't go to bed hungry—that, too, will keep you awake. A snack high in complex carbohydrates helps lull you to sleep.

Some women first experience sleeplessness at menopause when blood levels of calcium, magnesium, and the amino acid tryptophan decrease. The Center for Climacteric Studies recommends supplements of these nutrients for insomnia. Tryptophan supplements are no longer on the market, but the amino acid is present in carrots, beets, celery, spinach, alfalfa, turkey, and milk.

A soak in a hot tub is a great way to loosen tension and prepare you for sleep. A handful of one or more of the herbs mentioned in the next section will help waft you to dreamland.

Herbal and Folk Remedies

FRAGRANT VALERIAN, the original source of the tranquilizer Valium, has been used as a tranquilizer and soporific since antiquity. The "fragrance" is actually rather disgusting, so you will no doubt prefer to take the herb in capsule or tincture form—both are sold in health food stores.

A BEDTIME drink made by steeping a teaspoon each of passionflower (used in some over-the-counter preparations) and skullcap is sure to make you sleepy. Other tranquilizing herbs include lemon balm, catnip, lady's slipper root, peach leaf, birch leaf, hawthorn, lavender, lettuce, and wild cherry bark.

IF AN alcoholic drink is your chosen nightcap, make it a glass of beer. The alcohol, malt, and hops are ancient tranquilizers. Early in this century, hops was an official remedy for delirium tremens.

THE SCENT of hops can make you drowsy. Add a handful to your warm bathwater, or use the blossoms to make hops pillows, an old-fashioned folk remedy. Sprinkle dried hops with alcohol and sew them into a pillow or sack. Refresh the pillow with new hops when they start smelling rank—

long exposure changes the chemical composition, releasing valeric acid, an odor you are unlikely to find pleasant unless you are a tomcat.

AFRICANS BOIL four or five dried orange leaves in a glass of water and drink the hot infusion with sugar.

A RUSSIAN insomnia remedy is hot milk and honey. In India, nutmeg is added. The tryptophan in the milk is an aid to sleep.

CHAMOMILE TEA has for centuries been a popular European remedy for a variety of common ailments, including sleeplessness.

WEST COAST Native Americans used the root of California poppy for sleep. The poppy contains chemicals similar to opium.

A PUERTO RICAN insomnia remedy: peel and cut up a fresh papaya, put it in a blender with a cup of milk. Add ice or refrigerate before drinking.

Jet Lag

To accustom your biological clock to the new time zone, rest in a quiet, darkened room at bedtime even if you are not tired. Don't nap, especially if your new bedtime is earlier.

Starting the day with gentle exercise gets you accustomed to activity at a new hour and loosens muscles so you are better able to relax and sleep later.

Eat at the mealtimes of the new time zone even if you are not hungry. Breakfast and lunch should be high-protein, low-carbohydrate. The last meal of your day should be low-protein, high in complex carbohydrates (fruit, vegetables, and grains).

When you fly from the East Coast to the West Coast, where the time is earlier, don't try to stay up three hours later your first night; go to bed at your usual time. After a good night's sleep, you should be able to adjust to the later hour the next night.

Pain

You could say that pain is nature's way of getting our attention in order to warn us of an environmental danger, such as fire or poison, or a personal one, such as disease or injury. The nature and intensity of pain seem to vary with the individual. Once you know what caused the pain, you can figure out how to get rid of it. For more about pain, see also page 150, PAIN MANAGEMENT, in the section on SPORTS INJURIES.

Our bodies produce painkillers in the form of endorphins. These natural chemicals are similar to opiates, which in the plant world are unsurpassed at dulling the sensation of pain. Exercise releases endorphins, so keep active to raise your pain threshold.

Pain caused by inflammation and swelling can usually be subdued by ice, rest, and anti-inflammatory medication. Physiatrist Howard Liss advises: If you have arthritis or any inflammatory condition that makes it painful to exercise, raise your anti-inflammatory blood level by taking aspirin or other nonsteroid the day before. Dr. Suzanne Gosselin points out that "regular use, even sporadically, of aspirin and other nonsteroid anti-inflammatory drugs, has been linked with adverse affects on joints. For example, NSAIDs can contribute to the breakdown of collagen, a constituent of joint cartilage." German chamomile is an excellent anti-inflammatory, and unless you are allergic to ragweed, a botanical relative, you can partake freely of this soothing herb. Feverfew and ginger teas are also anti-inflammatory.

Muscle and joint pains usually respond to heat, which stimulates blood flow to the area, softening and loosening tense muscle and cartilage.

Some people are turning to meditation as a means of coping with intractable pain by quieting the mind and hence the nervous system.

Our response to pain is to tense the muscles, which usually makes pain worse. The American Chronic Pain Association advises relaxation techniques to control how your body feels. An Asian strategy is to lie or sit quietly and note the character of the pain. Do not try to avoid the sensation; instead, mentally detach yourself from it, as if the pain existed as a separate entity.

In correspondence with the newsletter of the American Chronic Pain Association, various members claim good results from the following strategies: drinking distilled or spring water, bicycle-riding, stretching exercises, a vegetarian diet, and sleeping on a water bed or other special mattress. Group support is also considered important. (See the RESOURCES section at the back of the book for information.)

Herbal and Folk Remedies

....

ANALGESICS RELIEVE pain by blocking sensory nerves or depressing the central nervous system. Examples of herbal analgesics include teas made with wintergreen, meadowsweet, willow bark, poplar, valerian, skullcap, passionflower, lady's slipper root; and oils of rose, peppermint, wintergreen, and clove applied externally.

ANTISPASMODICS EASE the contractions that cause cramps and muscle spasms. Herbalists recommend dill, imperial masterwort, peppermint, angelica, valerian, lady's-mantle, pasqueflower, passionflower, skullcap, and chamomile.

IN PUERTO RICO, allspice is used externally as an anesthetic.

SHOSHONE INDIANS boiled the leaves, twigs, and stems of sagebrush and drank the tea for general aches and pains.

Stress

Coping with stress
Suzanne Gosselin, B.S.N./D.C., a Rockport, Massachusetts,
chiropractor, offers this advice:

- Modern life is stressful, and there is no quick or easy remedy for that. What we need to do is take personal inventory to see what we must change. There should be a balance between work and play, exercise and inactivity. Do we allow time for personal interests and growth? Developing different sides of ourselves helps keep us in balance.

- We find stressors in all categories: physical, chemical, emotional, spiritual, and environmental. These diverse stressors affect our bodies in the same way—they create muscle tension. There is a considerable amount of data on the mind-body connection and how it affects every cell.

- All sensory input—physical, emotional, or chemical—is processed by the thalamus, that portion of the brain which is affected by the limbic system. The limbic system is associated with emotions and sense of well-being. Because the limbic system and thalamus work so closely together, stress can affect the muscular system, resulting in constant contraction of muscle. Prolonged, unrelieved muscle tension can result in a cascade of metabolic activities that lead to a pain-spasm-pain cycle.

- We often think of muscles as the fairly large skeletal muscles that provide movement. Remember that there is a muscular component to the digestive system; our blood vessels are lined with muscles that control their opening and closing; and the diaphragm is a large muscle at the base of our lungs that regulates the rate and ease of our breathing.

- Good nutrition provides the building blocks for health at the cellular level. Diet is a tool for coping with stress as well as medical problems. If we don't eat properly, our glands, especially the adrenals, don't get what they need to cope with stressors and keep our bodies in balance.

- Junk food taxes the system with chemical stress. Caffeine, white sugar, alcohol, and tobacco are also chemical stressors.

- Physical activity is a positive way to relieve stress. It helps you relax,

produces endorphins, increases circulation, brings vital nutrients to your cells, and facilitates the removal of toxins, which are chemical stressors.

- Too often we stress strength and neglect flexibility. To relieve and manage tension, find some form of stretching exercise. We can't do enough stretching. Yoga is excellent, as well as some forms of aerobic exercise such as golf, dancing, or tai chi that encourage flexibility.

- Physical stressors: think about what you do daily that aggravates your muscle structure. Your posture: do you walk tall, stand and sit straight, and avoid slouching? What about your sleeping position? We think that when we sleep our bodies are relaxed. This is a misconception. If our muscles are out of neutral position, they tense and even go into spasm. Many people get a good quantity of sleep, but not good quality. They wake up stiff, sore, or with a headache. Your spine should be in a straight line, your pillow supporting your head in neutral position. Sleeping on your stomach stresses your lower back and neck.

Make friends. Researchers have discovered that people who have a strong support network tend to be healthier, both physically and psychically.

Don't repress your emotions—let them out. Bottling up your feelings leads to tension and possibly physical ailments over time.

Recognize your personal sources of stress and how they affect you. Keeping a diary is a helpful tool.

People often feel stressed by what seem to be overwhelming responsibilities and/or difficulties. Learning and developing problem-solving strategies helps reduce stress by making your responsibilities and difficulties manageable.

Sometimes we bite off more than we can chew in terms of commitments and responsibilities. Learn to say no.

Many people become stressed and impatient while standing in line, sitting in a doctor or dentist office, and so on. Bring a book or notebook or find something to do while waiting—it helps pass the time.

Don't overschedule your time. Rushing from one appointment or task to another allows you no time to unwind.

Be sure to get enough rest. People who are short of sleep usually grow short of temper and are generally more stressed out. Take short breaks during the day, especially if your work is physically repetitious, and leave yourself some time for play in the evenings and on weekends.

Breathing deeply can help you relax and expel toxins.

Certain vitamins and minerals can help you cope with stress: try to take B vitamins, vitamin C, and 400 to 1,000 milligrams magnesium daily.

The Ears and Eyes:

From Ear Infections to Sties

The relationship between these sense organs is not only geographical; they constitute our most important sources of information about the world. A diet rich in vitamin C, which is abundant in fresh, raw fruits and vegetables, helps you build immunity against infections. Vitamin A and beta carotene aid night vision, protect against oxidation, and help keep mucous membranes moist and supple. Leafy greens and yellow vegetables and fruits provide the carotene your body needs to manufacture vitamin A; liver and cod liver oil are excellent sources of vitamin A.

EAR PROBLEMS

Your ear is a complex mechanism, consisting of delicate passageways, membranes, bones, tubes, fluids, and nerves that transmit sound and maintain your equilibrium. Your **outer ear,** the visible portion, includes the opening to the hourglass-shaped canal leading to your eardrum. Your **middle ear** contains the eardrum and surrounding bones and air spaces. Your **eustachian tube** connects the back of your nose and middle-ear space. Your **inner ear** houses nerve endings for the organs of hearing and balance.

Melissa S. Pashcow, M.D., F.A.C.S., Associate Attending in the Department of Otolaryngology at New York Eye and Ear Infirmary and Clinical Instructor in Otolaryngology at New York Medical College, New York City, reminds us: "Nothing smaller than your elbow should be put into your ear! Your ear canal lining is extremely delicate. To avoid scratching the skin surface and courting infection, do not poke or probe your ears."

Ear Infections

Treating an external ear infection
Advice from Dr. Melissa Pashcow:

- Most bacteria cannot live in an acid environment. Acidifying your ear canal by instilling drops of diluted vinegar can be helpful. (See directions below.) I sometimes recommend Burow's Solution, a 2 percent solution containing vinegar, available in pharmacies.

- Alcohol drops also kills fungus and bacteria that cause ear infections. If your eardrums are intact, you could apply eardrops composed of equal parts vinegar and alcohol. However, alcohol in irritated or infected ears can cause a painful burning sensation.

- To instill eardrops: (1) wash your hands and tilt your head to one side so the ear being treated faces up. (2) Pull your earlobe up and back and instill the recommended number of drops, being careful not to touch your ear with the dropper. (3) Leave your head tilted for three minutes. You can wipe away excess medication with a tissue, and gently place cotton in your ear.

- Some earaches actually originate in the jaw, triggered by TMJ, an inflamed temporomandibular joint. A warm wet washcloth or other warm compress should give you some relief.

Middle-Ear Infection

Ear infections are frequently a complication of colds or flu. They are caused by bacteria that spread from inflamed nasal membrane or a sore throat to your middle ear, causing infected fluid (or pus) to build up behind your eardrum. The main symptom is an earache and a feeling of pressure and blockage in your ear. Hearing may be muffled, and you may have a fever, nausea, and vertigo. If symptoms persist more than a day or two, see a doctor immediately. Ear infections can lead to serious complications, including loss of hearing.

Treat a sore throat promptly: the infection can spread to your eustachian tubes. When you have a cold or flu, blow your nose by holding one nostril and expelling gently.

An allergy attack can lead to ear discomfort via an inflamed eustachian tube. Avoiding allergens and controlling your environment may help. For example, smoking and being exposed to tobacco smoke may contribute to ear discomfort.

A well-balanced, low-fat diet may help you resist ear infections.

Herbal and Folk Remedies

A UNIVERSAL folk remedy for earache is rest, a few drops of olive, sesame, or safflower oil to soften the earwax, and the application of warm compresses or a heating pad to ease the pain. Adding crushed garlic to oil before dropping it in the ear also kills bacteria. In the Middle East, lemon juice is dropped in the ear to provide the acid environment that would kill bacteria.

THE USE of onions as an antiseptic for ear infections is ancient and universal. In some cultures, an onion is baked or roasted and, when it has cooled to body temperature, attached to the outside of the ear with tape or a bandage. Russians boil the onion for five minutes, squeeze it, and put both juice and pulp in the ear. Warm mashed garlic, papaya, and pumpkin have also been used similarly in various folk medicines.

THE WINNEBAGO Indians boiled the entire yarrow plant, then used the warm tea as eardrops.

HERBALIST JETHRO Kloss advises soaking your feet in a hot footbath with a tablespoon of mustard added; applying a poultice made with slippery elm, an herb available in health food stores; or sipping tea made with oregano. If an ear abscess breaks, he advises washing out your ear with warm peroxide.

MANY HERBALISTS advise drinking echinacea or goldenseal herbal tea and/or eating raw garlic to support your immune system and heal the infection.

Ear Pain While Flying

As the plane ascends, free air in your middle ear expands, causing your eardrum to bend outward. As the plane descends, cabin pressure increases, pushing your eardrum inward. On both occasions, chewing and swallowing forces air in and out of your eustachian canal, relieving the pressure.

Advice from the American Academy of Otolaryngology on relieving ear pain while airborne:

- Chewing gum or mints causes you to swallow more often, thus relieving ear pressure. Don't sleep while the plane descends because you may not swallow frequently enough.

- Yawning is an even better than swallowing because it activates the muscle that opens your eustachian tube.

- If neither of these measures works, try to pop your ears by pinching your nostrils, shutting your mouth, and gently expelling air into your closed mouth.

- To avoid ear infection or damage, don't fly when an upper respiratory infection or allergy clogs your air passages. If air travel is unavoidable, use a decongestant spray or drops an hour or so before the plane is to land, and don't blow your nose—it forces mucus into the eustachian tubes.

Earwax

Earwax is produced in the outer part of your ear canal where it repels water and traps sand and dust particles before they reach your eardrum.

Removing earwax
Advice from Dr. Melissa Pashcow:

- Earwax is made up of dead skin, oil, and sweat. Ordinarily, you don't have to remove it—as a protective mechanism, your ear cleans itself. Wax is constantly renewing and pushing the old wax to the opening of your ear canal. Probing your ear with a Q-Tip is like ramming gunpowder into a cannon—you drive the wax up against your eardrum and can injure the ear canal skin or possibly even rupture your eardrum.

- You can soften the wax with a few drops of warm peroxide or mineral oil. Be sure the solution is at body temperature—substances that are too cold or too hot can affect the structures in your ear that maintain equilibrium, and make you dizzy.

- You can buy over-the-counter ear-cleaning kits, but before you use one, be sure that your problem really is accumulated wax. You could have a blocked eustachian tube or an ear disease or disorder. Diabetics and people with small, bony growths in their ears must be particularly cautious. If you have a perforated eardrum, do not put any of these over-the-counter products in your ear, as they may cause an infection.

Insects in the Ear

The American Academy of Otolaryngology states that gnats, moths, and cockroaches are the insects most likely to get in your ears. Gnats can get trapped in the earwax; the larger insects cannot turn around or back out.

The academy advises flushing your ear with warm water using a bulb syringe. After removing the gnat, apply alcohol drops to dry out your ear and prevent infection. Larger insects can be immobilized by filling your ear with mineral oil. To avoid ear injury, have a doctor remove the insect.

Itchy Ears

According to the American Academy of Otolaryngology, itchy ears are most often caused by chronic dermatitis, a skin inflammation. The academy recommends decreasing your intake of greasy foods, chocolate, sugar, and starches, which can aggravate the condition.

Short-term itching can also be caused by a fungus. Dr. Melissa Pashcow recommends alcohol drops after you swim or shower, but only if you have "healthy ears." Instilling alcohol into an irritated or infected ear canal can cause burning and/or pain. If you don't have an ear dropper, Dr. Pashcow suggests improvising one from a drinking straw cut into one-thirds. Put one end of the straw in the alcohol, and capillary action will draw the alcohol up into it. Use this straw as a medicine dropper to apply the alcohol to your external ear canal opening. Do not put the straw into your ear canal.

Folk and Herbal Remedies

ALOE VERA gel soothes itching and kills any fungal or bacterial infection that may be causing it. Simply apply a little fresh or bottled gel to the itchy spot with your finger. (If you use a live plant, cut off a portion of the leaf, split it, and scrape out the gel.)

OATMEAL IS a traditional remedy for skin itching and irritation. Make a tepid solution by placing a cup of oatmeal in a clean sock or other cloth and steeping it in a basin of lukewarm water until the oatmeal is dissolved. Dip a washcloth in the solution and bathe your ear with it.

Ménière's Syndrome

A chronic ear problem possibly caused by fluid buildup in the inner ear, Ménière's syndrome is somewhat unpredictable in the way it comes and goes. A typical attack lasts twenty minutes or so. Symptoms include a ringing or buzzing sound in the ears, fluctuating hearing loss, pain and sensation of pressure in the ears, and intermittent nausea, vomiting, vertigo, and balance problems. There may be sweating and pallor. Sometimes Ménière's sufferers fall or feel drunk.

Coping with inner-ear balance disorders
The Vestibular Disorders Association has this advice:

- Your inner-ear fluid is influenced by certain substances in your blood and other body fluids. To provide stable body/fluid blood levels so fluctuations in inner-ear fluid can be avoided, eat approximately the same amount of food at each meal, and don't skip meals. Distribute your fluid intake evenly throughout the day. Limit your intake of sugar, salt, and alcohol, and avoid caffeine, aspirin, MSG, and tobacco.

- Some inner ear disorders can be aggravated by allergies. Stress and fatigue can trigger an attack, so rest and relax as much as possible.

- If vertigo attacks you without warning, don't drive, swim, or climb ladders.

A high level of salt or fatty acids in the blood is believed to be a factor in Ménière's syndrome. Regular aerobic exercise has been shown to reduce fatty acids.

To relieve nausea, chew a pea-sized piece of fresh gingerroot. You can also take $1/2$ teaspoon dried or one teaspoon fresh ginger in tea.

Swimmer's Ear

Swimming, showering, shampooing, and humidity can result in an infection of the outer-ear canal sometimes called swimmer's ear. Water trapped in your ear can make the skin soggy and vulnerable to infection from a fungus or bacteria. Your ear will feel blocked and probably itch. As the infection progresses, your ear canal becomes swollen and leaks a milky fluid. The cartilage in front of your ear canal feels tender, and you may have swollen glands.

Swimmer's ear

Advice from the American Academy of Otolaryngology:

- Drop mineral or baby oil in your ear before you swim or shampoo.

- After you swim or shower, tip your head from side to side to allow each ear to drain. Squeeze a medicine dropper of alcohol or equal parts

white vinegar and alcohol into your ear. Wriggle your ear so it is thoroughly washed with the solution, then tilt your head to drain the ear. Alcohol helps dry the ear, and, along with vinegar, kills bacteria and fungi.

Tinnitus

A ringing or buzzing in your ears can be the result of hearing loss due to aging or noise damage, a diet high in saturated fats, low blood sugar, or a reaction to smoking, caffeine, aspirin, or certain prescription drugs.

Learning to cope with tinnitus

Advice from otolaryngologist Melissa Pashcow:

- Your inner ear has only one artery, so many diseases affect the ear. If tinnitus affects your sleep, turn on a clock radio or a white noise machine at bedtime to drown out the noise. If you still have trouble sleeping, it is okay to take an antihistamine occasionally.

- If you have high-frequency hearing loss or work around noisy equipment, wear earplugs. Get the spongy type that conform to your ears—not the more brittle earplugs that break off in your ear. If your professional occupation subjects you to constant noise, wear heavy-duty earmuff-like protectors.

Dr. Donald J. Brown, a Seattle physician writing in Let's Live *magazine has these suggestions:*

- Reduce your consumption of sugar, simple carbohydrates, and saturated fats, and increase your consumption of complex carbohydrates, fiber, and protein.

- To keep your blood sugar level constant, eat small, frequent meals instead of three large ones.

- Avoid stress when possible, and practice strategies for coping with it (see pages 169 to 171 in Chapter Seven, "The Nervous System").

- Ginkgo leaf tincture is said to improve circulation to the brain and

relieve tinnitus. Cayenne pepper also stimulates circulation.

EYE PROBLEMS

The structure of your eye is somewhat like a camera. The lens focuses viewed objects on your retina; the iris opens and closes like a camera shutter to regulate the amount of light that enters your eye; and the retina, which lies in back of the eye, functions as the film, conveying the image to your brain via the optic nerve. Not only do your eyes give you essential information about the environment, they also reveal the presence of diabetes, glaucoma, and other chronic diseases.

Our ability to focus on close objects gradually declines from childhood—hence the need for reading glasses or bifocals after we reach the age of forty. Certain eye diseases, such as cataracts and macular degeneration, are usually age-related. Genetics is often a factor, says Maria Arnett, M.D., Ophthalmologist and Associate Attending Physician at Beth Israel Medical Center in New York City and New York Eye and Ear Infirmary.

Bags under the Eyes

Excess skin under your eyes or on your upper lids is partly genetic, says ophthalmologist Debra S. Guthrie, M.D., Attending in Ophthalmology at New York Eye and Ear Infirmary, Beth Israel Medical Center, and New York Downtown Hospital in New York City. When the skin under your eyes loses elasticity and sags, you appear to have pouches under your eyes. It helps, says Dr. Guthrie, to drink lots of water, sleep on two pillows, and apply cool compresses.

Bloodshot Eyes

Sun, wind, smoke and other irritants, eyestrain, and heavy alcohol consumption can tinge your eye red or make blood vessels visible. This happens when the tiny blood vessels that line our eyes get dilated, says Dr. Debra Guthrie. She recommends cool compresses applied for five or ten minutes every hour or two to help shrink the blood vessels and restore normal color.

Over-the-counter remedies that "get the red out" exacerbate the problem, Dr. Guthrie warns. You can get addicted to the vasoconstrictor so that your eyes don't clear unless you use it. If you insist on using these preparations, do so for no longer than three days. People with glaucoma should never use the eyedrops unless they are approved by their ophthalmologist.

Black Eyes

A black eye is a bruise surrounding your eye. The recommended treatment is crushed ice, compresses, or anything cold applied for five or ten minutes as often as can be tolerated. For more information, see page 219 in Chapter Ten, "Emergencies."

The bones around your eye protect it from injury, says Dr. Debra Guthrie, but you do need to see an ophthalmologist to make sure there is no internal damage. Meanwhile, to avoid bruising, it's important to treat your eye immediately. To decrease the swelling around your eye more quickly, she advises, be sure your head is elevated above your heart. If you need to lie down, prop up your head on a couple of pillows.

Blepharitis

The name may be unfamiliar, but you may recognize the symptoms: irritation, burning, and sometimes a red eye. The irritation is frequently caused by overactive oil glands along the eyelids combined with bacterial byproducts at the base of the eyelashes. Dandruff-like particles form along the lashes and eyelid rims. According to the American Academy of Ophthalmology, the condition frequently occurs in people who have oily skin, dandruff, or dry eyes.

The American Academy of Ophthalmology recommends warm compresses twice a day. Dr. Debra Guthrie recommends following the compress application with gentle massage of the oil glands along your eyelids to normalize the environment. Next, she says, you should thoroughly cleanse the lids and lashes with a solution composed of two or three ounces warm water and three drops baby shampoo. Gently scrub your eyelids for two minutes, using a cotton ball, then rinse thoroughly with your eyes closed and discard leftover cleaning solution.

Cataracts

The term "cataract" comes from a Greek word meaning waterfall and refers to the cataract sufferer's sensation of viewing the world through a curtain of water. Associated with aging, a cataract is a thickening of the eye lens, gradually reducing vision. Surgically removing a cataract is usually a safe and simple procedure.

The condition may be caused by faulty nutrition, a metabolism problem, or a reaction to certain drugs such as steroids. Before microwave oven technology improved, radiation leaks from the oven were thought to be a factor.

The Center for Science in the Public Interest notes that researchers have not yet established a cause, but data show that oxidation of lens protein is highly correlated with cataracts. Current thinking points to sunlight's ultraviolet rays oxidizing the lens protein, thereby ruining the crystalline structure of the lens so that either the protein crystals clump together or water seeps in and scatters incoming light. As protection against ultraviolet rays, wear a hat with a wide brim and sunglasses with UV protection even on overcast days.

Genetics often determine whether a cataract will form, but smoking hastens the process, says Dr. Debra Guthrie. Certain medications, metabolic processes, and trauma are contributing factors. She advises a diet rich in antioxidant vitamins C, E, and A as a possible preventative.

Shopping for sunglasses?

Advice from the American Academy of Ophthalmology:

Studies show that people who spend long hours in the sun without adequate eye protection have an increased chance of developing eye disease.

- For everyday wear, choose lenses that are medium to dark gray, uniformly shaded, and impact-resistant. Check the label to make sure the lens blocks at least 99 percent of ultraviolet (UV) light. Large, close-fitting, wraparound frames protect your eyes from radiation that may enter from the sides.

- When buying nonprescription sunglasses, hold them at a comfortable distance and, with one eye closed, look through the lens at a regular pattern such as a floor tile. Move the glasses from side to side and up and down. If the lines wiggle, try another pair of glasses.

- Sunglasses with the best UV absorption, optical quality, and breakage resistance don't have to be expensive. Studies show that the best sunglasses cost no more than $1.50 more than the worst.

Folk and Herbal Remedies

BATHE YOUR eyes three or four times daily with a tepid solution made with ¼ teaspoon each rue and comfrey in a cup of boiling distilled water. **Warning:** Boil the water for ten minutes first to remove impurities and discard any homemade eyewash after twenty-four hours.

APPLY A poultice of softened eyebright (*Euphrasia officinalis*) and fennel in equal parts and a dash of mace, and drink a tea made with the same ingredients.

Conjunctivitis

Conjunctivitis is an inflammation of the conjunctiva, the tissue that lines your inner eyelids and sheaths the globe of your eye. Your eyelids burn, smart, and redden; your vision becomes very sensitive to light; pus forms; and your eyes are crusted shut in the morning. Pinkeye, where the eyeball becomes reddish, is a common form of conjunctivitis.

The infection is highly contagious, so don't share the towels, pillows, or washcloths of an infected person or spread the infection by sharing yours. Eye makeup can also harbor disease organisms, so get rid of any you have used when your eyes were infected.

Preventing and controlling conjunctivitis
Advice from Dr. Maria Arnett:

- A well-balanced diet rich in vitamins A and E helps you maintain healthy eyes.

- Eye infections can be spread by handshakes and touching objects an infected person has handled. It helps to wash your hands frequently and keep your fingers away from your eyes.

- There are many types of conjunctivitis—viral, bacterial, and chemical. Each requires a different treatment. For this reason, you should see an ophthalmologist. In addition to any treatment your doctor may prescribe, you may find it helpful to apply warm compresses for five minutes three or four times a day.

Advice from Dr. Debra Guthrie:

- Itching is the classic symptom of conjunctivitis, which can be a reaction to an allergen such as eye makeup or an infection.

- Try warm compresses dipped in a boric acid solution.

- If you experience severe pain or blurred vision, or the skin around your eye is inflamed, see a doctor at once. You should also see a doctor if your symptoms haven't improved after three days.

Preventing infections from contact lenses

Drs. James V. Aquavella, Herbert E. Kaufman, and R. D. Richards, writing in Patient Care, *a trade publication for physicians, offer this advice to contact lens wearers:*

- Extended-wear lenses should be replaced every six months and removed and cleaned at least once a week. Use sterile commercial saline preparations for soaking the lenses.

- Bathroom humidity breeds germs. Store your lenses and paraphernalia in the bedroom or other non-humid place. Use two lens cases and alternate them every week. One should be sun-dried while the other is in use.

- To keep your lenses scrupulously clean, wash your hands before handling or inserting a lens, and never put a lens in your mouth.

Herbal and Folk Remedies

AT THE first sign of conjunctivitis, take vitamin A supplements or cod liver oil—in this way you may be able to head off an infection.

MAKE A strong goldenseal solution—two teaspoons to a cup of boiled water—and use it for warm compresses. Apply for fifteen to twenty minutes three times a day.

FOLLOW THE instructions above, using turmeric instead of goldenseal.

APPLY COMPRESSES made with equal parts of eyebright (*Euphrasia officinalis*) and fennel or chamomile three times a day, and drink tea made with these ingredients at the same time.

Dry Eyes

A sensation of grittiness or sticking are symptoms of dry eyes. Usually this is caused by decreased tear production as one grows older, but dry eyes can result from a medical disorder, or be a reaction to certain medications or smoking marijuana.

Coping with dry eyes
Ophthalmologist Debra Guthrie offers this advice:

- Your eyes may feel gritty, or you may feel as if you have rocks in your eye. Profuse tearing is also a symptom of dry eyes.

- Your tears are composed of water, mucus, and oil. Produced by tiny glands on the rims of your eyelids, the oil slows the evaporation of tears. When there is not enough oil in your tears, dry eyes can result. If the release of oil is blocked, your eyelids feel heavy and uncomfortable. To stimulate production and release of the oil, gently massage your eyelids.

- Although you may feel as if an eye bath would relieve the condition, don't rinse your eyes with plain water because you will rinse away the natural oils.

- Preservatives in artificial tears may irritate your eyes, so use these drops no more than three times a day. You can buy artificial tears without preservatives, but they're considerably more expensive.

- Winter air, which has little moisture, forced-air heating, and air-conditioning can exacerbate dry eyes. In winter it helps to set containers of water on top or at the base of your radiators to humidify the air.

Naturopath Dr. Lucy Smith at the Natural Health Clinic of Bastyr University in Seattle, Washington, recommends an eyewash made with boric acid. As a preventative, she advises a diet that includes plenty of oil and antioxidants such as vitamins C and E.

Dry eyes can be caused by abnormalities in the structure of the eyelid that make tears evaporate quickly, or by blinking abnormalities. Japanese researchers have discovered that people blink three times less often when looking at a computer monitor than they do when reading books.

Smoking and tobacco smoke, aspartame sweeteners, alcohol, and certain drugs such as some antibiotics, diuretics, pain relievers, and tranquilizers can aggravate dry eyes, so avoid them when they are not necessary treatment for a disease.

Eyestrain

Blurred vision at the end of the day, a burning sensation, and/or a bifrontal headache are all symptoms of eyestrain.

All of our muscles work in pairs, Dr. Debra Guthrie reminds us. A slight misalignment of your eye muscles combined with poor lighting can strain your eyes. Eyestrain, says Dr. Guthrie, can also result from a small refractive error in the structure of your eye, which is not noticeable until you are spending long hours at a computer terminal or doing close work. You may need corrective lenses, or a new prescription for them.

If you sit at a video display terminal, the top of the screen should be at or slightly below eye level. A copy holder attached to the side of the screen requires fewer head and eye movements and changes of focus. Dr. Maria Arnett recommends a glare screen for the computer. If you are reading, working at a computer terminal, sewing, or doing other close work, Dr. Arnett advises, rest your eyes every hour or so by closing them or gazing at something distant for five minutes.

Blinking is a brief respite that spreads a film of tears over your eyes. When you stare at a computer terminal, says Dr. Guthrie, your blink reflex slows down. This is particularly true for contact lens wearers. It helps to use eyedrops and remember to blink frequently.

Glare can contribute to eyestrain. Read with the light behind you, Dr. Guthrie advises. A 15 percent tint in your reading glasses may be helpful, she says, especially when reading glossy magazines that reflect light. Incandescent or full-spectrum lighting is better than fluorescent lighting, but since that is what most work places provide, you may have to bring a lamp and provide your own.

Both physicians recommend seeing an ophthalmologist if your eyestrain doesn't improve.

Advice to older adults who may be particularly sensitive to glare
Professor Robert Rosenberg, O.D., Professor of Optometry at State University of New York College of Optometry in New York City, and clinical consultant for Lighthouse Low Vision Services, suggests:

- Avoid extremes of lighting contrast. Have only one light source in a work area. This light should be as far as possible from your usual line of sight so as to be outside your visual field.

- The strongest light in a room should be directly on your task, but the surrounding area should also be well lighted at one-third to one-fifth the brightness of your work area. Lighting in the rest of the room may be even less, but at least one-tenth to one-fifteenth as bright.

- Don't use the luminous ceiling type of lighting because you can never get the light source out of your visual field. If the room has a lot of ceiling lights, wear a visor.

- Move desks, TV, and other furniture out of bright light. Don't watch TV in the dark.

- When outdoors, shield your eyes with a broad-brimmed hat as well as sunglasses.

Itchy or Irritated Eyes

People with allergies are the ones who suffer most often from itching and irritation, especially during hay fever season or when air pollution levels are high. Eyestrain can also make your eyes feel irritated and sometimes itchy.

Wearing goggles and/or wraparound sunglasses outdoors and air-conditioning your bedroom help you avoid allergens.

Chlorine can be irritating, so wear goggles when you swim in chlorinated pools. Goggles also help protect you if you apply chemical sprays to your lawn or garden. A better strategy would be not to use chemicals. However, even natural pesticides can be irritating if you are sensitive to them.

Ophthalmologist Dr. Maria Arnett recommends cold compresses for five minutes three or four times a day to relieve itching.

Macular Degeneration

The macula is a small area on your retina that allows you to see fine details clearly. As they age, many people experience blurring or a dark area in the center of their vision. According to the American Academy of Ophthalmology, normal chemical reactions from light in the eye activate oxygen, which may cause macular damage. Some experts believe that overexposure to blue radiation from sunlight contributes to macular degeneration. They advise sunglasses with an orange or amber tint that absorb most blue radiation, all ultraviolet radiation, and block 75 to 90 percent of visible light. Dr. Maria Arnett says that it is essential to wear sunglasses year-round to protect your eyes from ultraviolet radiation in direct sunlight as well as reflections from water, snow, and ice. Glasses also protect your eyes from the drying effects of wind.

Macular degeneration has become an important issue, observes ophthalmologist Dr. Debra Guthrie, because people are living longer. It seems to happen more often to people who are lightly pigmented or farsighted, she says. There have been no good studies, she adds, but anecdotal stories indicate that antioxidant vitamin supplements may be helpful in slowing down the progress of macular degeneration.

In a University of Chicago study, researchers discovered that a daily carrot or other beta carotene-rich food reduces the likelihood of macular degeneration by 40 percent. **Note:** More beta carotene is released from cooked carrots. Dr. Arnett advises a well-balanced diet with supplements of vitamins A and E, zinc, and selenium.

The American Academy of Ophthalmology recommends checking your vision daily with an Amsler Grid like the one pictured below:

To use the grid, wear your reading glasses (if you wear them) and in good light, with one eye closed, hold the grid twelve to fifteen inches from your eyes. Gazing directly at the center dot, note whether any areas are blurred or distorted. If you observe any visual abnormality, see your doctor immediately.

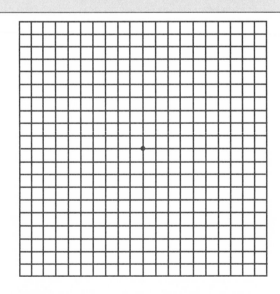

Night Vision

As we age, we become less able to discriminate the border between light and dark, and we adapt less quickly to different areas of brightness, notes Dr. Robert Rosenberg. He advises lots of vitamin A to alleviate night blindness.

During World War II, it was observed that pilots who snacked on bilberry jam were more successful at hitting targets at night. Used in European folk medicine for centuries, the bilberry is the European equivalent of the blueberry.

Puffy Eyes

Puffiness around the eyes comes from water retention, says Dr. Maria Arnett. A cold compress for about five minutes two or three times a day helps bring down the swelling. Some women like to make compresses with cold skim milk, Dr. Arnett says; others like to use cucumber slices.

Possible causes of and preventatives for puffy eyes
Advice from ophthalmologist Dr. Debra Guthrie:

- We have no fat around our eyes to act as a water barrier, so when we eat very salty foods, then sleep horizontally, excess fluids settle around the eyes. This often happens after we eat Chinese food containing monosodium glutamate (MSG). Sometimes aging is a factor. As we get older, the membrane that holds back the fat cushioning at the back of our eyes becomes stretched, so the fat slides forward.

- Sleeping on several pillows prevents fluid or fats from settling around the eyes and reduces puffiness. **Note:** This position may aggravate back problems.

- Use cold, wet tea bags as compresses. The coldness and the tannic acid reduce swelling.

Spots and Floaters

Spots or cobwebs floating across your vision field are usually harmless. What you are seeing is shadows on your retina cast by small clumps of protein that have become trapped in fluid inside your eye. Although everyone has them, few people notice the floaters until middle age. They require no treatment, advises Dr. Maria Arnett. However, if the spots suddenly appear or increase in size or number, you could have a serious vision problem and should see a doctor immediately.

Sties

A pimple filled with pus, a sty is caused by an infection of the hair follicle on the eyelash, states Dr. Debra Guthrie. Applying warm compresses three or four times a day will bring the sty to a head.

Oiliness in the eyelashes is a contributing factor, says Dr. Maria Arnett. If you are prone to sties, she advises, wash your eyelashes when you wash your face. Using a Q-Tip dipped in baby shampoo diluted 50 percent with water, be sure to clean the base of your lashes.

Most sties are actually chalazions, observes Dr. Guthrie. These are lumps caused by plugged oil glands. A warm compress applied for five or ten minutes three or four times daily, followed by a gentle massage of the oil glands, should help remove the plug.

9

The Skin and Hair:

From Abscesses to Thinning Hair

Our largest and most sensitive organ, the skin is our main defense against pollution, disease, and climatic extremes. Antimicrobial secretions and beneficial bacteria provide a barrier against harmful bacteria and viruses; sweat and oil glands flush out wastes and toxins.

No keeper of secrets, the skin proclaims our emotional weathers and physical well-being. In some sensitive people, the skin may betray a recent chocolate, sweets, or fried foods binge; it is usually the first bodily organ to show signs of illness or aging.

Another indication of how well we treat ourselves is our protective mantle of hair, composed mostly of protein and, like skin, slightly acid in chemical composition.

Abscesses and Boils

An abscess is a swollen, inflamed area of tissue filled with pus or infected material, most often caused by streptococci or staphylococci germs. The area will be red, swollen, and tender. If the wall of the abscess breaks down, the abscess bursts. An abscess can occur any place on your body, but most often appears in the groin, armpit, or other hairy location.

We tend to think of boils as being smaller than abscesses; however, Dr. Robin Ashinoff, Chief of Dermatologic and Laser Surgery at New York University Medical Center in New York City, notes that a boil is simply the lay term for an abscess. Dr. Ashinoff advises soaking the abscess with warm compresses for fifteen minutes every hour until it drains.

Herbal and Folk Remedies

HERBALISTS CONSIDER boils and abscesses to be a sign of "impure" or "polluted" blood. The typical treatment is to prescribe an herb classified as an alterative—a substance that stimulates the elimination of toxins and gradually alters the course of a disease. Examples of alteratives are burdock root, chickweed, dandelion, dogwood, ginseng, goldenseal, yellow dock, sarsaparilla, wild Oregon grape, spikenard, blue flag, cleavers, nettles, and red clover.

TO MAKE tea with one of these herbs, steep a teaspoonful of the leaves in a cup of boiling water for ten minutes; boil roots the same length of time. Along with the alterative, a mild laxative such as asparagus, boneset, borage, licorice, burdock root, hibiscus, apples, cucumber, prunes, figs, or psyllium seeds may be prescribed to assist your body further in eliminating toxins.

APPLY A hot goldenseal compress (one teaspoon to $^1/_2$ cup boiling water) at least three times a day. Herbalists recommend that you drink a cup of goldenseal tea or swallow a capsule at the same time you apply it externally.

AFRICANS HEAT the crushed fruit of a papaya, wrap it in a clean cloth, and apply, still warm, to the abscess. This poultice is kept in place with a bandage until the inflammation subsides and the swelling goes down.

A POLISH remedy is to soak a piece of white bread in warm milk and apply to the area. Both ingredients are drying, helping to "draw" the infection.

A SCOTTISH remedy is to drink a wineglass of water with a quarter teaspoon of Epsom salts dissolved in it. Epsom salts are an old-fashioned laxative and a method of getting rid of toxins.

TEA TREE oil is recommended for a variety of skin infections because it is antiseptic. At the same time that you apply the oil externally, you could drink a few drops in a cup of hot water.

Acne

Heredity has a great deal to do with whether or not you get acne, a common skin problem for young adults, characterized by pimples and blackheads. Some women suffer acne before their menstrual periods or at menopause. Excessive oil secretion, microbial infections, and glandular disturbances are the main causes; stress can be a contributing factor. Formerly, chocolate and a high-sugar diet were considered culprits, but recent research has exonerated them.

To combat acne, increase your intake of fresh fruits and vegetables. They are rich in vitamin C, which helps you resist infection. Leafy greens, yellow squash, and broccoli are high in beta carotene, a nutrient essential for healthy skin. At the same time, decrease your consumption of fats and sugars—they won't improve your complexion. And stay away from greasy hair products, cautions Dr. Robin Ashinoff—they can trigger an attack.

Herbal and Folk Remedies

ALTHOUGH MAINSTREAM medicine considers the value of such practices questionable, an alternative healer would recommend improving your digestion and cleansing your system of toxins by taking one or more of the alteratives listed under ABSCESS in this chapter.

IN DAYS of yore, people took spring tonics to purify their blood of all the rich and greasy food eaten over the winter. Sulfur and molasses is probably the most famous one. Made with two tablespoonfuls sulfur and one cup molasses, this old-fashioned Scottish blood purifier supposedly prevents spots and pimples.

AN EXTERNAL application of a cut fresh garlic clove, a bruised cabbage leaf, or a 5 percent concentration of tea tree oil may help clear up infection and inflammation. Test these substances on the inside of your wrist to be sure you are not sensitive to them before you apply directly to the inflamed area.

IN HER article on home remedies in *Parade* magazine, writer Joan F. Hamburg reports that cosmetic mogul Adrien Arpel makes homemade pimple cream by adding a pinch of alum to 1/4 cup witch hazel. Apply the paste to your face and let it dry. You can use it under makeup.

Age Spots

These are dark patches of pigmentation, sometimes raised above the skin surface, and most often seen on the face and hands or any areas that are constantly exposed to sun. They are also called liver spots.

Like freckles, age spots are your skin's response to sun damage, says Dr. Robin Ashinoff. Over-the-counter bleaching agents don't do much good, she adds. You could try alpha hydroxy acids or lemon juice, but either can irritate or make you sensitive to sunlight.

According to an Australian study, age spots can be reduced by wearing sunscreen and hats.

Herbal and Folk Remedy

JAMAICANS USE a cold infusion of sinicle Bible, also called "leaf of life"—
a big, green desert plant. Keep the plant in water and drink the juice for
internal cleansing, to clear liver spots on your skin.

Athlete's Foot

Actually a form of ringworm, this stubborn fungus infection attacks you between the toes, causing the skin to become red, itchy, and raw or cracked.
Like its botanical relative the mushroom, the athlete's foot fungus loves
warm, damp, and dark environments. What better home could there be than
the dark interior of a shoe and a sweat-soaked sock?

To discourage such unwelcome flora or to prevent the infection
from spreading, keep your feet and your socks scrupulously clean and dry.
A peroxide wash helps discourage bacteria. Wear natural-fiber shoes that allow ventilation, and wool or cotton socks that absorb perspiration. Spend as
much time as possible barefoot or in sandals to keep your skin dry.

Soaking your feet in a solution of strong tea—either plain old supermarket variety, or herbal tea with a high tannin content such as bearberry
or oak bark—discourages perspiration. Sprinkling talcum powder on your
feet helps absorb moisture.

Herbal and Folk Remedies

A 5 PERCENT solution of tea tree oil, available in health food stores, is a
good fungicide.

YOU COULD also try a mixture of half water, half aloe vera gel—fresh, if
possible. In laboratory studies, aloe has also proved effective in combating
athlete's foot.

TO DRY up the rash and soothe itching, apply a baking soda paste.

Blackheads and Enlarged Pores

Treating blackheads
Advice from dermatologist Dr. Robin Ashinoff:

- People with large pores are more prone to blackheads. If you do get blackheads, leave them alone—don't try to squeeze them or pick at them. The dark color is not dirt but melanin, a skin pigment that appears black.

- Bleaching agents such as lemon juice or alpha hydroxy acids may have some effect on the appearance of your skin, but they can irritate and may make you more sensitive to sunlight.

- Applying ice or astringents to your skin contracts the blood vessels and temporarily changes the appearance of your skin: the pores will appear smaller.

Herbal and Folk Remedies

THE BLOSSOMS of the elder tree have been used for centuries to soothe, soften, and whiten skin. Make a strong tea by steeping a tablespoon of the blossoms for ten minutes in a cup of boiling water.

TO TEMPORARILY shrink large pores, splash on an astringent using the above proportions and one of these astringent herbs: rose petals, comfrey, bay leaf, yarrow, sage, nettles, strawberry leaves, raspberry leaves, or horsetail. For a quick astringent, splash on distilled witch hazel or split a leaf of fresh aloe and apply the gel.

Blisters

See BLISTERS, pages 220-221 in Chapter Ten, "Emergencies."

Body Odor

Perspiration evaporating on your skin is your body's way of cooling you down when you are overheated. Cotton, wool, and other natural fabrics wick moisture away from your skin, while synthetic fabrics can leave you steaming in an airtight barrier of chemical odors.

Your diet can be detected in the odor of your sweat. Meat-eaters have stronger body odors than vegetarians; green plants are rich in chlorophyll, nature's deodorant.

Controlling body odor
Advice from Dr. Robin Ashinoff:

- Body odor is caused by bacteria. Bathe with an antibacterial soap and make sure to launder your clothing frequently.

- If skin areas perspire excessively, bathe them once a day in freshly brewed tea—the tannic acid is astringent and helps arrest perspiration.

Herbal and Folk Remedies

FOR A soak to control perspiration, you could also use tea made with a highly astringent herb such as oak bark, bearberry leaves, witch hazel, or tormentil.

A VINEGAR soak (one tablespoon cider vinegar to one quart warm water) once or twice a day may help control odor.

FRESH ALOE, which is antibacterial, is used in some "natural" deodorants. Cut a leaf and rub the gel over the skin area you wish to deodorize. **Warning:** Test the aloe on a small, tender skin area such as your inner arm to be sure you won't have an allergic reaction.

Bruises

Bruises most often result from injury, sometimes from a circulatory problem, and more rarely from certain diseases where the blood does not clot. They are caused by broken capillaries that bleed under the skin. Initially they are blue or purple, then fade to green and/or yellow.

If you bruise easily, increasing your intake of vitamin C can help strengthen capillary walls. The best way to get this vitamin is to eat raw fruits and vegetables. In fruits and vegetables, vitamin C is accompanied by substances such as bioflavenoids that help your body absorb and utilize this vitamin efficiently.

Avoid aspirin and other anti-inflammatory drugs that interfere with clotting. Estrogen and steroids can also contribute to bruising.

When you are injured, ice the area to reduce pain and swelling and arrest bleeding. It is important that this be done immediately after the injury. Once the bruise appears, folk medicine won't help. For more information, see pages 219–220 in Chapter Ten, "Emergencies."

Herbal and Folk Remedies

APPLY A cold compress for twenty minutes two or three times daily using a strong tea made from one or more of the following herbs: arnica, bay leaf, comfrey, violet, marigold, balm of Gilead, St. John's wort, oregano, and blue iris. You can also make a compress using cold distilled witch hazel.

AN EASTERN European remedy is to apply raw egg white to the bruise.

Chapping and Windburn

Cold, windy weather can make your skin redden and crack. This is particularly true for people with sensitive skin and those who spend a great deal of time out of doors. People who must frequently wash their hands or plunge them in water are likely to suffer from red, roughened skin that may be cracked and sore.

Preventing chapped skin
Advice from dermatologist Dr. Robin Ashinoff:

- To prevent chapped lips, use lip balm with sunscreen and lick your lips as seldom as possible.

- Dry, cracked skin around your mouth can be an allergy to oral dentifrices— toothpastes, mouthwashes, and liquid plaque preventatives may be irritating your skin. Eliminate or change your present product and see if there's an improvement.

Herbal and Folk Remedies

TO AVOID chapped lips, apply glycerin—it softens your lips and prevents them from cracking.

TO AVOID chapped hands, rub them with table salt after they have been in water, then rinse in cool water and dry.

BAG BALM, lanolin, or a mixture of aloa vera gel and olive oil will ease chapping and roughness, especially if the oiled skin is protected with rubber gloves.

EQUAL PARTS of rosewater and glycerin make an old-fashioned hand lotion that is very soothing and softening.

RUB YOUR hands with an herbal oil prepared by steeping two tablespoons dried herbs in $^1/_2$ cup olive or vegetable oil in a sunny window for two or three weeks. Marigold and comfrey soothe irritated skin; elder and lime blossoms soften and whiten; mint and chamomile are antiseptic and healing; marshmallow root and Irish moss soften.

Dandruff

Dandruff flakes are not a form of dry skin but an infection caused by an organism similar to yeast.

Coping with dandruff
Advice from dermatologist Dr. Robin Ashinoff:

- Wash your hair every day with coal tar or salicylic acid shampoo, but be aware that the coal tar may discolor white or gray hair.

- Excessive dandruff may actually be scalp psoriasis, which should be checked out by your doctor.

Herbal and Folk Remedies

WHEN YOU shampoo, apply a strong tea made with rosemary as a final rinse.

JAMAICANS RUB fresh aloe vera gel into the scalp. The gel has been shown to be effective against fungi and bacteria.

AFRICANS BURN papaya leaves and rub the scalp with the ashes.

Dry Hair

Exposure to sun, salt water, or alkaline shampoos can dry your hair. Other predisposing factors are genetics, the aging process, and the environment. The remedies listed under DULL HAIR, later in this chapter, are also helpful for dry hair.

Herbal and Folk Remedies

···

APPLY OLIVE or corn oil to your scalp and hair. Dark-haired people can add cappuccino, French roast, or espresso coffee to the oil. Cover with a shower cap and leave overnight, or apply hot towels to your oiled hair for an hour or so.

TO GET the benefit of both oil and egg, use real egg mayonnaise instead of vegetable oil.

Dry Skin

Some people are genetically predisposed to dry skin, which ranges from a sensation of tightness to a papery texture and dry flakes. Dry skin can also be due to environmental factors (winter winds and cold or arid indoor air), diet, or aging. Although it is a problem for only some younger adults, dry skin is common after menopause when estrogen declines and your oil glands function less vigorously.

Drink plenty of water or herb tea to hydrate body tissues. Include in your daily diet at least a tablespoonful of monosaturated vegetable oil such as olive, avocado, or canola, and liberal portions of leafy greens, broccoli, squash, apricots, cantaloupe, and other foods high in vitamin A.

Certain environmental factors can dry both skin and hair. Avoid prolonged exposure to sunlight unless you use sunblock. Steam heat and air-conditioning contribute to dry skin unless moisture in the air is replenished. Containers of water set on radiators, a simmering teakettle, a vaporizer, cut green leaves set in bowls of water, and houseplants add humidity.

Replace moisture by misting your face with water several times a day—a perfume atomizer works well. Avoid alkaline and glycerine-based soaps; instead, use cold cream or vegetable oil as a face cleanser followed by a vinegar rinse to restore the pH balance (1 tablespoon cider vinegar to one quart warm water). For overall moisturizing, take baths instead of showers. Use soap only where necessary.

To add moisture to your skin, Dr. Robin Ashinoff recommends Crisco or similar vegetable shortening. It is very emollient, she says, and has no preservatives.

Herbal and Folk Remedies

STEAMING DISLODGES dirt, cleans the pores, stimulates circulation, and moisturizes. Cover your head with a towel and lean over a basin of steaming water to which a handful of peppermint leaves, orange blossoms, rosemary, chamomile, thyme, rose leaves, or rose hips has been added. **Warning:** Don't lean too close—steam can burn!

REMOVE DEAD, flaky skin once a week by scrubbing with ground almonds or apricot seeds, dry oatmeal, bran, fine cornmeal, wheat germ, or brewer's yeast, or a face mask of mashed papaya.

AN INFUSION of orange blossoms or rose petals (remove the astringent white heel), chamomile, or comfrey can be used as a moisturizing skin freshener. Steep one tablespoon dried or two tablespoons fresh blossoms or leaves in one cup boiling water for ten minutes, cool, and splash on your face.

COCOA BUTTER, clarified butter, lanolin, petroleum jelly, and olive, safflower, and apricot oils are excellent moisturizers. Apply immediately after cleansing, while your skin is still warm. Wait about fifteen minutes before applying makeup to allow skin to absorb the oil, then tissue off excess. For best results, apply before taking a bath—steam helps your skin absorb moisture.

AFRICANS USE papaya blossoms infused in oil as a skin smoother.

A TRADITIONAL Eastern European dry skin remedy is to make a face mask with raw, grated carrot. An updated version, easier to handle, is to cook the carrots until slightly softened, puree in an electric blender, and apply to your skin. It is said to improve elasticity and smooth wrinkles.

FOR OVERALL skin care, chamomile is popular in Europe. Soak in a warm tub to which a handful of chamomile flowers or a tablespoon of the oil has been added. **Warning:** Chamomile is botanically related to ragweed, so if you are allergic to the latter, you may be sensitive to chamomile as well.

HERBAL OILS are good to have on hand to use either straight from the bottle or as a base for homemade hand cream. Add two tablespoons dried herb to $\frac{1}{2}$ cup safflower, sunflower, or almond oil, pour into a clear glass jar, cover, and set on a sunny windowsill to steep for two or three weeks, then strain. Marigold and comfrey are healing to chapped and irritated skin; elder or lime blossoms whiten and soften; mint and chamomile are antiseptic and healing; marshmallow root and Irish moss soften the skin.

TO MAKE hand lotion, add one teaspoon beeswax, $\frac{1}{4}$ teaspoon honey, and a pinch of gum benzoin to a cup of the herbal oil, heat in an enamel or glass saucepan until the wax is melted, then whip the mixture until creamy.

WRINKLES CAN be minimized by massaging your skin with any of the oils listed above. To smooth away crow's-feet, massage the area at the corner of your outer eyelids in tiny, counterclockwise circles for one minute a day. Wrinkles in the lower part of the face can be treated by using the same motion on the area of your chin below the incisors. For forehead wrinkles, place your fingers just above your eyebrows, in line with your pupils, and massage in a clockwise motion.

Dull Hair

Putting the shine back in your hair can be as simple as changing your shampoo. Some are too alkaline and upset the normal pH balance of your hair, which is normally slightly acidic. Aging, which slows down oil production, can result in dry, dull hair.

Dr. Robin Ashinoff recommends frequent shampooing. Don't use conditioner, she says. It may build up on your hair and dull it.

> ## The following remedies are used in Eastern Europe to give hair strength and life:
>
> - Mix one egg yolk, two teaspoons kerosene, and one teaspoon lemon juice. Work the mixture into your hair, leave on for fifteen minutes, and wash off.
>
> - Wash your hair with fresh birch sap.
>
> - Massage rosemary oil into your scalp every day. (Rosemary oil or tea is also used in folk medicine to darken gray hair.)

Herbal and Folk Remedies

TO RESTORE the acid balance of your hair and remove soap residue, add a tablespoon cider vinegar to a quart of warm water and use it for your final rinse.

TO BRING out highlights, make a strong herbal tea by steeping either rosemary (for brunettes), chamomile (for blondes), or henna (for redheads) in a cup of boiling water; cool and use for a final rinse.

EGG YOLK adds shine to your hair. Add a whole raw egg to your usual shampoo or shampoo with only a whole raw egg.

Eczema

Often caused by allergies and sometimes triggered by stress, eczema can be either a temporary flare-up or a chronic skin problem. Symptoms include itching, redness, crusting, scaling, and serum-filled blisters. A general term that applies to a variety of skin conditions, both dry and moist, eczema can be a response to something you ingest (dairy products are often the source) or touch (household detergents are a frequent source of contact dermatitis, a form of eczema). Predisposing factors include a persistent fungal or bacterial infection of the skin.

Controlling eczema
Advice from dermatologist Dr. Robin Ashinoff:

- Eczema is the worst type of dry skin. To conserve moisture, bathe less in winter. Instead, take quick, cool showers. Use a non-soap cleanser such as Cetaphil.

- If you have eczema on your hands, wear cotton-lined rubber gloves when you wash dishes. At bedtime, coat your hands with petroleum jelly and wear gloves.

- Crisco or similar vegetable shortening is a good moisturizer because it is very emollient and contains no preservatives.

Certain foods may aggravate eczema, including citrus fruits, cheese, eggs, milk, nuts, fish, wheat, red meats, fermented foods such as vinegar and soy sauce, alcohol, frozen, canned, or otherwise processed foods, and food additives. See if your condition improves when you eliminate these items from your diet for two months. Gradually add the foods again, one at a time, eliminating any that cause an eczema flare-up. In this way, you may be able to assume a normal diet, eliminating only the foods that trigger your allergic reaction.

Avoid dust and air pollution—each can trigger an allergic reaction.

Prolonged sweating, immersion in water, exposure to irritating substances or extreme heat or cold, or prolonged sun exposure are predisposing factors.

Wear natural-fiber clothing—chemicals in synthetic fibers can irritate.

Be sure your diet includes foods rich in beta carotene (green and deep yellow vegetables), vitamin E (whole grains, especially wheat germ), vitamin C (fresh, raw produce), and quercetin (red wine, broccoli, summer squash, shallots, and onions).

Herbal and Folk Remedies

A DIET rich in B vitamins, corn oil, and lecithin (at least 4 grams daily) helps clear up eczema. In some studies, oil of primrose capsules—500 milligrams six to eight times a day—has proved effective in controlling eczema. Drinking a mixture of beet, celery, and tomato juice ($^1/_4$ cup each) two or three times daily may also be helpful.

HERBALIST JETHRO Kloss, author of *Back to Eden,* a very influential book about herbalism and natural healing, recommends equal parts of burdock root, yellow dock, yarrow, and marshmallow. Steep a teaspoonful of this mixture in a cup of boiling water. Drink $\frac{1}{2}$ cup four or five times a day, and wash the affected parts with it.

TRY CHAMOMILE poultices, which are anti-inflammatory. Comfrey poultices help heal lesions. The herb contains allantoin, a natural chemical that stimulates cell renewal. To soothe itchy, sore outbreaks, try buttermilk compresses. In India, a poultice or compress of marijuana leaves is used to treat eczema and other skin problems.

CHAMOMILE OR oat or rye bran added to bathwater is very soothing.

TO HELP soothe inflammation, take the herb heartsease internally in tea and externally in medicated oil made by steeping two tablespoons dried herb in $\frac{1}{2}$ cup olive oil for two weeks.

THE HERB feverfew acts as an antihistamine. Steep one teaspoonful of the dry leaves in a cup of boiling water for ten minutes and sip it once a day. At least three times a day apply feverfew compresses made with two teaspoonful feverfew steeped in a cup of boiling water. **Note:** Test for sensitivity to this herb by first applying it to a small patch of skin.

TANNIC ACID helps dry up blisters. At least three times a day use tea bags or tea compresses. Herbs with a high tannic acid content include oak bark and bearberry leaves.

APPLY APPLE cider vinegar to the lesions.

GOLDENSEAL ROOT and gotu kola leaves are excellent for all sorts of skin problems. Sprinkle on the powdered herb or use medicated oil or butter made by gently heating two tablespoons of the dried herb with 2 cups oil or butter for about 15 minutes.

FRESH ALOE vera gel is both soothing and healing to a variety of skin problems, including eczema.

BORIC ACID ointment, sold in pharmacies, has been recommended at least since the turn of the century.

EXPERIMENTERS HAVE found that echinacea salve, made with a combination of fresh root, leaves, and flowers, is very healing to eczema.

Herpes Simplex
(Cold Sores)

Herpes simplex is a skin infection caused by the herpes virus. The most visible symptom is sore, itchy blisters filled with clear fluid around the lips or genitals. Much of the time, the infection is dormant. When active, it is highly contagious. Herpes can be activated by fever, sunlight, menstruation, pregnancy, and other factors.

Herbal and Folk Remedies

MASH A mango, spread on a cloth, and use as a poultice two or three times a day. In a Chinese study, two chemicals in tropical mangoes were effective at inhibiting multiplication of herpes simplex virus.

IN ANOTHER study, a salve made from the roots, leaves, and flowers of fresh echinacea plants healed herpes inflammation.

YOU COULD also try eucalyptus oil, which is antiseptic.

Lice

Your most likely way of getting lice is from your school-age child. The insects or their eggs are readily transferred when children share combs, brushes, or headwear. The main symptom of lice is itching; you also may feel as if something is crawling through your hair.

Dr. Robin Ashinoff recommends an over-the-counter pyrethrin preparation such as RID. In order to get rid of lice, you must kill the eggs (nits) as well as the lice. Dr. Ashinoff advises that you wash all clothing and bedclothing as well as anything that might come in contact with your hair in soap and very hot or boiling water. Some people add Lysol to the wash water to help kill the nits.

Herbal and Folk Remedies

··

IN TOBACCO-GROWING areas, tobacco leaves are sometimes used to repel or kill insects because nicotine is a powerful insecticide. Africans boil fresh tobacco leaves to use as a hair and head wash two or three times a day.

TO KILL nits, which often remain even after an insecticide is used, comb tea tree oil, which is antiseptic, through your hair.

BEFORE OVER-THE-COUNTER preparations for killing lice appeared, people applied kerosene to their hair, let it sit for a few minutes, then shampooed several times.

Psoriasis

Psoriasis appears on the skin as flat, symmetrical, reddish brown spots or plaques covered with silvery white scales. Rapidly maturing cells move to the skin surface, where they collect, forming red patches covered with scaly white dead cells, most often seen on the elbows, scalp, lower back, and upper chest. It is possible to have only a temporary bout with psoriasis, but usually the condition is chronic. Little is known about its possible causes.

Exposure to sunshine can help clear up psoriasis in its early stages. According to the Rodale Press editors, Omega 3 oils can inhibit cellular production of leukotrienes, which trigger itching and scaling. Eat purslane or tuna fish, mackerel, and other oily fish, or take fish oil supplements. Some people find it helpful to eliminate meats from their diet.

Controlling psoriasis
Some tips from the American Academy of Dermatology:

- Go easy on the alcohol; drinking impairs recovery.

- Beta blockers can irritate your psoriasis. If you are taking this medication and your psoriasis worsens, you may want to discuss alternative medication with your doctor.

- Avoid spices, wine, nuts, and brandy.

- Use milk products, especially yogurt and cottage cheese; sauerkraut; and pickles.

- A rice diet is helpful. Cook ten ounces of dry rice and eat it with fresh or preserved fruit for your daily quota.

- Treat vaginal infections promptly because they can aggravate the condition.

- Applications of Avon's Skin So Soft works for some people.

- To slow the rate of cell multiplication, apply heat with a hot water bottle or heating pad at a few degrees above body temperature to the inflamed area.

- Take supplements of vitamins B2 and B6.

- Light mineral oil keeps the area moisturized.

Some tips from the National Psoriasis Foundation:

- Take 1,800 milligrams or ten capsules of fish oil daily.

- For scalp psoriasis, rub your scalp with olive oil or vegetable oil, cover overnight with a shower cap, then wash with coal tar shampoo. (Coal tar preparations make your skin sensitive to sunlight, so take precautions. They can also discolor gray or light hair.) For best results, shampoo often, cleansing carefully and rinsing thoroughly.

- To remove scales and moisturize skin, shower daily with cool water and mild, nonalkaline soap—Dove has tested mildest. Rinse thoroughly to avoid soap residue. Apply oil to your skin before you towel off, then pat your skin dry gently—don't scrub.

Apply moisturizer again in the morning or evening, depending on when you last showered. To remove grime, use baby oil rather than abrasive hand soaps.

- Exposure to sunlight is a recommended psoriasis treatment; but be sure to wear sunscreen—sunburn can be devastating. Keep your hair as short as possible so your scalp benefits from the healing effects of summer sun. If you are taking photosensitizing drugs for psoriasis, however, stay out of the sun completely.

- Avoid dry skin, exposure to irritants and harsh weather, and tomato sauce and spicy foods.

- The psoriasis medication psoralen can make you feel nauseous or dizzy if you take it on an empty stomach or with a meal containing fatty foods.

- Topical applications of vitamin D3 and oral doses of vitamin D may give relief; coal-tar-based bath products or skin creams can soothe an outbreak; oatmeal baths can control itching. Cream that contains 0.025 percent capsaicin from hot peppers relieves itching; after a month of regular applications, all symptoms improve. Before you apply medicines to your skin, remove the scales with water.

- Keep your weight down.

- It is not known whether smoking actually causes psoriasis, but it has been established that there's a link.

- The following can cause flare-ups or aggravate existing ones: throat infections, skin injuries and irritations, chronic friction in any skin area, shaving with a rusty razor, diarrhea (which can cause flare-ups in the anal area), tight shoes, and ingrown toenails.

Herbal and Folk Remedies

IN INDIA, powdered gotu kola leaves provide the base for medicated oil or ghee (clarified butter): one ounce herb is gently heated in one pint oil or ghee and applied to the lesions.

THE HERB feverfew is antihistamine and anti-inflammatory. Apply compresses and drink the tea. Aloa vera, gotu kola, goldenseal, oak bark, sarsaparilla, or ordinary tea can be used similarly.

COMPRESSES OF white oak bark, high in astringent tannin, help dry up the sores.

Scars and Stretch Marks

Stretch marks are associated with pregnancy, but some people get them after weight loss. You can't really get rid of them, says Dr. Robin Ashinoff. To do so, you would have to change the elastic property of your skin.

Herbal and Folk Remedies

WHETHER OR not you get stretch marks is largely determined by genetics. However, in many cultures, a pregnant woman anoints her abdomen with oil or butter to soften the skin. Olive oil is often used. In the Caribbean, cocoa butter is applied. Vitamin E oil is also said to reduce scarring.

Shingles
(Herpes Zoster)

The scientific term comes from a Greek word meaning "belt." Shingles is a rash of blisters, usually on the trunk, which surrounds your body like a belt. Caused by a virus that affects the nerve roots in your spinal cord, the rash is accompanied by a burning sensation and sometimes pain. Initial symptoms include slight fever and loss of appetite. The average bout lasts from ten to fourteen days, but older people recover more slowly. Drugs are not usually required.

Cold compresses and analgesics such as aspirin soothe irritation.

Large doses of vitamins C and B12 may help, as may taking in extra calcium and magnesium, elements essential to the nervous system.

Some doctors recommend Vaseline Intensive Care lotion for post-herpatic neuralgia.

You may get relief by using Zostrix, a preparation that contains capsaicin extracted from cayenne pepper. Capsaicin relieves pain by stimulating, then depleting, substance P, released by the nerve endings and thought to be responsible for pain.

Thinning Hair

Thinning hair and bald patches are more often male problems, but women do experience thinning hair after an illness, anesthesia, or menopause, or because of genetic predisposition.

Herbal and Folk Remedies

···

HERBAL PREPARATIONS that are reputed to restore hair include tinctures of arnica and southernwood, burdock root oil, and nettle tea.

MASSAGING YOUR scalp stimulates circulation; if you do this regularly, it may stimulate hair growth.

EDGAR CAYCE, a clairvoyant known as the "sleeping prophet," advised used motor oil rubbed into the scalp.

Warts

Warts, caused by a virus, are small, hard growths on the outer layer of skin.

Dr. Robin Ashinoff recommends a pumice stone to pare down the growths.

Journalist Catherine Clifford reports that dermatologist Dr. Jerome Z. Litt, instructor at Cleveland's Case Western Reserve University School of Medicine, has an unusual cure for warts around the fingernails: apply four layers of adhesive tape in alternating layers, making an airtight but not irritating package. Leave on for six and a half days, leave off for a half day, then apply a new bandage for another six and a half days. Continue until the wart disappears, which may take from two to six weeks. He thinks the treatment may work because the tight bandage cuts off viral air supply.

High doses of vitamin C are also recommended.

Herbal and Folk Remedies

···

IN CHINA, dried sesame flowers are soaked in water for thirty minutes, then brought to a boil. The liquid is used as a wash for ten days.

APPLY TEA tree oil, effective against viruses.

APPLY LATEX from fresh greater celandine, dandelion, or fig; tincture of thuja, fresh aloe vera or garlic, raw potato or green walnuts.

Emergencies:

From Abrasions to Sunburn

Some injuries and illnesses happen at hours and places when medical assistance is not readily available. A few, such as arterial bleeding or certain eye injuries, demand immediate treatment before you set off for the emergency room. Others, such as cuts and bee stings, can usually be treated at home. Much of the information in this chapter comes from an interview with Dr. Karen Lawson, family practice physician currently working in the Emergency Department at Unity Hospital in Minneapolis, Minnesota.

Abrasions

Abrasions most often result from falls where we slide and scrape the skin on an elbow, knee, hand, or other landing point.

Treating abrasions
Advice from emergency room physician Dr. Karen Lawson:

- When you scrape your skin, dirt may become embedded in the wound and cause scarring. To avoid scars, you may have to really scrub the area to get the abrasion clean. (If this is not possible, see a doctor.) Soak the area in water and Betadine, Epsom salts, Ivory soap, or Woolite. Keep the injury clean and dry for the next twenty-four hours.

- There is a possibility of tetanus infection with any abrasion, burn, cut, puncture, wound, or injury that breaks the skin surface. If it is ten years or more since you had a tetanus shot, you should get one within seventy-two hours.

After the injury is cleaned, don't apply a bandage—let the air get to it so the abrasion can dry.

Herbal and Folk Remedies

SPRINKLE A coating of myrrh over the wound. This powdered resin, sold in health food and herb stores, is antiseptic, speeds healing, and seems to prevent scarring.

THE HERB comfrey, which is sold in herb shops and health food stores, contains allantoin, a natural chemical that speeds healing by stimulating the formation of new cells. After you clean the abrasion, moisten dried comfrey leaves with hot water, wrap in a sterile cloth, and apply to the wound. (Omit the hot water if you use fresh leaves.) Be sure the area is perfectly clean before you apply the comfrey, for allantoin regenerates the skin so quickly that new skin can form right over the dirt.

PETROLEUM JELLY applied after the wound is cleaned has been found to act as a protective shield and speeds healing.

Warning: Dr. Lawson cautions that occlusive (airtight) dressings such as petroleum jelly or a poultice should not be left on for more than a couple of hours. If any symptoms of infection, such as pus discharge or spreading redness, occur, seek medical attention immediately.

Bee Stings

If the bees always seem to find you, or if you are highly allergic to bee stings, prevention is essential. Bees are attracted to perfume, hair sprays, bright colors, and flowered prints, so you might want to avoid wearing them anyplace where you are likely to encounter a bee.

Apply ice or a cold pack to the area to reduce pain and swelling.

Mud for bee stings?
Dr. Karen Lawson has this advice:

- Mud, especially if it is clay-based, does draw out the sting and the stinger. However, in urban and suburban areas you do have to be careful, because there could be fecal contamination.

- A baking soda compress neutralizes the acidic bee serum. Because it is drying, the soda also soothes the sting and draws out the stinger.

- Wasp venom, however, is alkaline, so if you're stung by a wasp, apply vinegar to soothe it.

Herbal and Folk Remedies

IN HONDURAS, sliced raw garlic is rubbed over the sting to prevent irritation and swelling.

AN AFRICAN remedy is to apply the milky liquid of green papaya fruit. The stinger is said to come out by itself in a short time. The papain in the papaya breaks down the protein in the bee venom. Fresh papaya or even meat tenderizer, which contains papain, the active ingredient in papaya, may also work for you. To avoid irritation, be careful not to get the papaya juice in your eye.

RUB THE sting with crushed elderberry leaves or the milky-white juice of a milkweed pod. Elderberry is a traditional and universal remedy for skin irritation; the milkweed latex is useful in drawing out the stinger.

APPLY AMMONIA water, which is alkaline, to counteract the acidity of the bee venom.

Bites

Animal Bites

The chief hazards with animal bites are the possibility of infection, especially tetanus infection, and the danger of rabies. You are more likely to contract rabies from a wild animal in summer, but both wild and domestic animals can be rabid in other seasons.

Treating animal bites
Advice from Dr. Karen Lawson:

- If the wound is deep, you may have a tendon injury, which requires immediate medical attention.

- If the wound is relatively superficial, soak it in water and Betadine, apply antiseptic, and cover with a sterile dressing.

- Is the animal rabid? Question the owner of a domestic animal to find out the status of its rabies shots. If you cannot identify the owner, or if the animal is wild, notify animal control authorities. They will keep it indoors and under observation for ten days. If the animal is rabid, you will need a series of rabies shots.

- When did you last have a tetanus shot? If it's been ten years or more, you should get one within seventy-two hours.

- If the bite is deep—to the bone—you should be on antibiotics. All human bites require antibiotics because the human mouth contains the most germs of any mammal's mouth.

Mosquito Bites

To discourage mosquitoes, use baby oil as a repellent—mosquitoes don't like to put their feet in it.

If you do get bitten, apply ice to reduce inflammation and swelling, then dab on household ammonia, which is alkaline, to neutralize the acid serum.

Avoiding and treating mosquito bites
Advice from Dr. Karen Lawson:

- To avoid bites from mosquitoes and sand fleas, take one garlic capsule three times a day, or eat three cloves of garlic. The garlic secreted in your sweat is an excellent insect repellent. You could also take 100 milligrams of thiamine three times a day or 60 milligrams of zinc once a day.

- Mosquito venom has an anticoagulant chemical that causes an allergic reaction. Take an antihistamine or anti-inflammatory such as aspirin. Calamine lotion is soothing and drying; witch hazel can be cooling.

Black Eyes and Other Bruises

A blow to your body or face is likely to result in a bruise. The skin discoloration at the site of the bruise is caused by tiny blood vessels that leak under the skin. If you bruise very easily, you may have a vitamin C deficiency. This vitamin, which is plentiful in fresh, raw fruits and vegetables, helps strengthen your capillary walls so you are less vulnerable to bruising.

Dr. Maria Arnett, Associate Attending Physician at Beth Israel Medical Center in New York City, recommends applying anything cold, preferably ice, as often as can be tolerated. Cold constricts your blood vessels and stops bleeding. Wrap ice in a cloth or towel before applying.

What about raw steak for a black eye?
Advice from Dr. Lawson:

- Raw steak is simply a malleable cold compress. For the first couple of days, cold is useful in reducing pain and swelling.

- After the bruise appears, home remedies don't do much good. It will be about a week before the bruise fades.

- Don't take aspirin for pain. The anticoagulant action causes more blood to leak under the skin, and the bruise will spread. To relieve discomfort, take acetaminophen.

- Vitamin C, zinc, and the bioflavonoids found in citrus fruits help you heal faster.

Blisters

A bad sunburn, a second-degree burn, or friction can produce blisters. You may be able to keep a burn from blistering by prompt application of fresh aloe vera gel. To cushion your skin against friction, wear work gloves when handling tools, and two pairs of socks—thin cotton inside, thicker wool outside—when you go hiking or walk long distances. A layer of moleskin over pressure points also gives you protection.

Treating blisters
Advice from Dr. Karen Lawson:

- A blister acts as a sterile dressing. You don't need to break the blister; your body will absorb the fluid.

- If the blister is on your feet or any area that gets a lot of friction, you could drain it with a sterile tool such as a needle. Clean the needle with peroxide or pass it through a flame. If you use fire to sterilize it, wipe the instrument clean of carbon so you won't contaminate the wound. Make as small an opening as possible, soak the blister in Betadine and water, and apply dressing. Check the blister daily. If the edges get red or there is pus or swelling, you may have an infection and should see a doctor.

Herbal and Folk Remedies

··

EASTERN EUROPEANS make a small opening in the blister, soak a piece of bread in milk and lay this "plaster" over the area. Dr. Lawson notes that this practice dates back to World War II. The milk and bread would help drain and dry the blister. In Europe, she said, rye may have been used because ergot, a fungus that grows on rye and often gets mixed in with this grain, has antibiotic properties. A wet tea bag will take the sting from fever blisters.

Burns

According to Dr. Karen Lawson, a first-degree burn is painful and red, but it doesn't blister. A second-degree burn is painful, red, and blistered, but you have sensation. Even second-degree burns can be treated at home unless you feel nauseous or the burns are on your face, the palms of your hands, or the soles of your feet. If the burn is large and you fear skin loss, or you can't clean the area yourself, Dr. Lawson advises emergency treatment. A third-degree burn is red, blistered, possibly charred, and there is no sensation. See a doctor immediately. Third-degree burns and large-area second-degree burns must be treated immediately because of the risk of scarring, infection, and even systemic dehydration due to water loss through the burn area.

Treating burns
Advice from Dr. Lawson:

- Tetanus infection is possible with second- and third-degree burns, so get a shot within seventy-two hours if you haven't had one in ten years.

- If you were burned by contact with something hot, plunge the injury into cold water to relieve pain and reduce swelling. Apply cold water, not ice, for ten minutes at ten-minute intervals.

- The gel from a fresh aloe plant is the best treatment for first-degree burns. It may sting second-degree burns. If you don't have aloe, apply vinegar.

- For pain relief, take two adult aspirin every four hours. **Warning:** Don't use aspirin if you're asthmatic or taking a blood-thinning medication.

- An intact blister is a perfect sterile bandage for a second-degree burn; don't break it. If it breaks by itself, rinse with cool water and apply a sterile dressing.

Dr. Robin Ashinoff, Chief of Dermatologic and Laser Surgery at New York University Medical Center in New York City, advises that there will be less scarring if you keep the burned skin clean and moist. She recommends an application of petroleum jelly, then covering the burn with a bandage.

Herbal and Folk Remedies

IN RUSSIA, hot-oil burns are treated with honey applied directly to the area. Dr. Lawson notes that honey is rich in B vitamins, which could help with skin regeneration. Although they are not recommended by most Western physicians, lubricants such as butter or olive oil are universal folk remedies.

MORMON TEA, a desert plant that can be found in health food stores, is high in tannin, which forms a protective coating over wounds. Native Americans used the powdered stems for burns. Ordinary tea that is brewed very strong—two or three tea bags steeped in boiling water for ten minutes—is also rich in tannin. You could also apply a wet tea bag directly to the skin.

Cuts and Wounds

Treating wounds
Advice from Dr. Karen Lawson:

- If the injury is on your face, especially if it is near or in your eye, cover it with a clean or sterile dressing and seek medical help immediately. Repairs to these areas may involve plastic surgery. The surgery must be done in the first couple of hours because after that time the edges of the wound start to draw together and an optimal repair might not be possible. A wound that is over $^1/_2$ inch long, or on your knuckle, knee, elbow, or other surface where continual bending would interfere with healing, also requires stitches.

- Examine the injury. Is it clean? Does blood ooze from the surface, or does it squirt? Squirting blood may indicate a cut artery. Get help immediately. Deep cuts that go to the bone and cuts that are $^1/_2$ inch or longer also require emergency treatment. If you haven't had a

tetanus shot for ten years or more, be sure to get one within seventy-two hours.

- Unless you're in the middle of the woods and have cut an artery, don't use a tourniquet. Apply local pressure above the wound, then ice, and elevate the wound.

- If you *are* in the middle of the woods or similar place where help is not immediately available, and you have cut an artery, apply the tourniquet to the part of your arm or leg that is closest to the trunk. Never put a tourniquet on your fingers or toes where the blood supply is tenuous.

- Small wounds should be soaked in water and Betadine, Epsom salts, Ivory soap, or Woolite. Keep the surface clean and dry for twenty-four hours so the scab can pull it together.

Dermatologist Dr. Robin Ashinoff advises that wounds heal better when they are washed with peroxide and covered with a bandage.

Herbal and Folk Remedies

CERTAIN HERBS contain substances that are very healing to cuts and wounds. It's not a bad idea to keep some in your kitchen, and to tuck one or two in your knapsack before you go camping:

COMFREY CONTAINS allantoin, a chemical that stimulates the manufacture of new cells. Moisten the dried herb with hot water, or bruise fresh leaves, wrap in a cloth, and lay over the wound. Herbalists caution you to be sure the wound is clean before applying comfrey because healing takes place so rapidly the wound may close over any debris left in it.

MYRRH IS a tree resin, best known to Christians as the incense the three Wise Men brought to baby Jesus. Powdered myrrh is antiseptic and very astringent—a potent healer. Sprinkle some on the surface of a cut, wound, or abrasion to dry up pus or blood. Keep the area dry by continuing to sprinkle on layers of myrrh. Don't apply a bandage—a scab should begin to form in a few hours.

THE POWDERED ROOT OF *GOLDENSEAL,* a woodland plant, was a favorite remedy of the Cherokee Indians, who used it for skin infections. Like myrrh, it is antiseptic and drying; apply it as you would myrrh. Both are sold in health food stores and herbal outlets. Use them individually or in equal parts for skin problems.

IF YOU are outdoors at the time of injury, there are a few wild plants it is helpful to know. Wild plant identification is not within the scope of this book, but you can buy wild plant identification guides in most bookstores and camping suppliers. *YARROW,* a botanical relative of the more familiar Queen Anne's lace, which it resembles, is a humble wildflower with a venerable history as a healing plant. During the Crusades, knights carried a few sprigs in their helmets to have available to stanch the flow of blood. Crush the plant and apply to the wound until it stops bleeding.

THE SPADE-shaped leaves of *PLANTAIN,* which grows in most lawns and dooryards, are such a common and familiar part of our surroundings most of us don't notice them. Once widely known as "soldier's herb," plantain is a blood coagulant that stops bleeding. Bruise the leaf to release its juices and lay the leaf over the wound.

SELF-HEAL (prunella vulgaris), also known as *HEAL-ALL,* or *WOUNDWORT,* is a modest member of the mint family with tiny purple flowers. You are likely to find it growing all over lawns and fields. The herb is astringent and rich in tannin. Boil some for a few minutes and use the tea to wash and help dry the wound.

IN PUERTO RICO, *EUCALYPTUS OIL* is applied to the wound as an antiseptic.

A JAMAICAN method of arresting blood flow is to wash the wound, squeeze on the juice of one lime, then apply the warm pulp of an ordinary green banana, and cover the whole with a bandage. In Africa, warm papaya pulp is used similarly.

TO STOP hemorrhaging, Africans wash papaya leaves and lay them over the cut or wound. Another African wound dressing is raw carrot cut in small pieces, wrapped in a cloth, and applied as a compress. To treat an infected wound, Africans wash the wound with soap and water, mash pieces of onion to extract the juice, then apply the juice to the wound.

Dizziness

The American Academy of Otolaryngology offers the following advice for preventing dizziness:

Dizziness is most often traced to a circulatory disorder. When your brain does not get enough blood, you feel light-headed. Everybody has felt dizzy on occasion after rising abruptly from lying down. Frequent dizziness may indicate a cardiovascular problem such as anemia, or a neurologic abnormality.

Certain drugs, especially stimulants such as caffeine and nicotine, can make you dizzy by decreasing blood flow to your brain. In some people, excess salt in the diet leads to circulatory disorders and dizziness.

Stress, anxiety, and tension can cause muscle tension and spasms anywhere in the body. When the spasms occur in the tiny muscle fibers lining your arteries, they can impair circulation and cause dizziness.

Motion sickness can make you feel dizzy.

Vertigo, a specific form of dizziness that disrupts your sense of balance, results from injury, infection, or allergy that affects your inner ear. Ménière's syndrome, an inner-ear disorder, also results in vertigo attacks. To reduce vertigo, avoid rapid changes in position and extreme or rapid head movements; reduce or learn to manage stress; avoid allergens; reduce or eliminate your intake of salt, sugar, fats, caffeine, and nicotine.

Stay away from ladders, dangerous equipment, and hazardous activities such as driving or swimming when you are dizzy or if you are prone to unexpected vertigo attacks.

When is dizziness critical?
Advice from Dr. Karen Lawson

- An episode of dizziness could indicate a crisis if you have history of a stroke, are diabetic and have eaten sugar, or high blood pressure has been diagnosed. You can also feel dizzy if you have been unable to eat and drink adequately or if you have a bleeding ulcer.

- If you feel better lying down, you could be suffering from dehydration and blood loss, perhaps from gastrointestinal bleeding or external injury.

- Older people who feel suddenly dizzy for no apparent reason should see a doctor immediately. Younger people could wait until the next day to consult a doctor if they have no significant health problems and are able to drink fluids.

- Use caution changing positions to avoid aggravating a possible low blood pressure problem.

- If the problem is Ménière's syndrome, a middle-ear infection, or motion sickness, you feel worse when you suddenly turn your head or move your eyes, or lie down flat. In this case, keep still and take an over-the-counter antihistamine.

Eye Injuries

Chemical in the Eye

If any chemical gets in your eye, it should be treated immediately, before you seek medical help, says ophthalmologist Dr. Maria Arnett, Associate Attending physician at Beth Israel Medical Center in New York City. Don't use an eyecup. Your eye should be flushed with running water or any nonacidic liquid for at least fifteen minutes. Stand in a shower, hold your head under a water faucet, or pour water over your eye. Keep the lids open and turn your head with the injured side downward to avoid contaminating your good eye. After you have flushed out the chemical, see your doctor immediately.

Cinder or Other Foreign Material in the Eye

If a speck of foreign material has gotten in your eye, it is most likely to be on the inner surface of your upper lid, or where the lid and the globe meet. You may be able to dislodge it by lifting your upper eyelid out and down over the lower lid.

If the globe of your eye is lacerated, cover it with a patch and seek medical treatment immediately. Don't eat or drink en route, as you may require anesthesia and surgery.

Ophthalmologist Dr. Maria Arnett warns that trying to remove foreign material from your eye with a Q-Tip, handkerchief, or other material could scratch the surface of your eyeball. To avoid this, Dr. Arnett recommends using natural or artificial tears to wash the speck into the inner corner of your eye, where you can remove it without irritation.

If You Are Hit in the Eye

For the first twenty-four hours, ophthalmologist Dr. Maria Arnett advises, apply ice wrapped in a cloth or towel for fifteen-minute periods as often as you can tolerate it. If your eye is hit by a small object that could damage the globe, or if the globe is red or your vision blurred, she strongly advises immediate medical treatment.

Fainting

Dr. Karen Lawson discusses fainting:

Even young, healthy people sometimes feel light-headed because of a sudden position change that causes an abrupt change in blood pressure. If you get up in the night to go to the bathroom, a reflexive drop in blood pressure may cause a fainting spell. This is more likely to happen to a male, however.

Remaining unconscious is your body's way of adjusting blood pressure. If you have a severe headache when you regain consciousness, your blood pressure could be very abnormal or you could have an intercranial injury. Get your feet higher than your head, drink water, and loosen your clothing. Seek help if the headache persists.

Fainting is also a classic symptom of early pregnancy.

Herbal and Folk Remedies

SIT DOWN and put your head between your knees.

A JAMAICAN remedy is to put a cool cloth on your face and a newspaper on your stomach.

Jellyfish Sting

Treating jellyfish stings
Advice from the Center for Medical Consumers in New York City, and J. E. Jelinek, M.D., Clinical Professor of Dermatology at New York University Medical Center:

Don't rub your skin or wash it with water. This activates toxins and promotes the formation of tiny cysts. To minimize the burning sensation, neutralize the toxin with vinegar, alcohol, or meat tenderizer. If hives or red welts appear, go to the emergency room immediately.

Mountain Sickness

Flatlanders who travel to Western mountain states often experience flu-like symptoms at elevations above 7,500 feet. This is more likely to happen if you are hiking. Symptoms may include headache, nausea, fatigue, insomnia, reduced urine output, and/or swelling of your hands, face, or feet. These symptoms are your body's response to decreased barometric pressure and oxygen supply. Your blood becomes more alkaline, altering your body's ability to exchange gases. Your lungs and brain retain fluid.

To reduce the possibility of mountain sickness, make altitude changes gradually to allow for acclimatization. Take it easy for the first few days until your body adjusts to the new altitude. When you are at high altitudes, drink plenty of fluid. While climbing, drink at least two quarts of water. Eat low-fat, high-carbohydrate meals and limit your intake of salt, alcohol, and caffeine.

Pronounced headache, lack of coordination, confusion, and severe nausea and vomiting indicate a life-threatening condition that should be treated immediately.

Nosebleed

Nasal bleeding can result from injury or illness. Recurrent nosebleeds may indicate a serious problem, so see your doctor.

Avoiding and treating nosebleed
Otolaryngologist Dr. Melissa Pashcow has this advice:

- Because your nasal membrane is very sensitive, it can dry out, crack, and bleed when the outdoor climate or indoor air is very dry. A saline nose spray helps to keep your nose moist. You can make this at home by mixing a teaspoon of salt in a cup of warm distilled water. A little petroleum jelly helps keep your nasal membrane moist. To avoid irritating sensitive tissue, apply it with your finger, not a Q-Tip. A third strategy is to moisturize the air with a humidifier or vaporizer.

- To stop the bleeding, sit with your head tilted forward slightly and squeeze your nostrils tightly shut for ten minutes without releasing your fingers. An ice pack on your nose and cheeks also stops bleeding. (Use frozen peas or cut-up vegetables if you don't have ice.)

- To prevent recurrent bleeding, do not blow blood clots from your nose; just gently wipe away any discharge.

- You can soften the crusts around your nose with vitamin A and D cream.

- If bleeding persists, see a doctor immediately.

Poison Ivy and Poison Oak

Both poison oak and poison ivy contain the allergen urushiol oil. If you know you have been exposed to this allergen, wash your skin immediately to get rid of the oil. Fels naphtha or similar household soap has been the traditional cleanser, probably because it dissolves oil, but rubbing alcohol or any soap will do; even plain water is better than nothing. To avoid reinfection, also scrub your clothing and any objects that have come in contact with your skin or the urushiol oil.

Dr. Robin Ashinoff recommends soaking the area in milk to soothe and cool the itch, followed by a topical application of aluminum sulfate. To reduce inflammation, she advises aspirin or Motrin.

Taking the itch out of poison oak and ivy
Advice from Dr. Karen Lawson:

- An oral over-the-counter antihistamine may prevent or reduce the rash.

- To help tame the itch and dry the blisters, soak in a lukewarm bath to which $1/2$ cup of baking soda has been added, then apply calamine lotion or zinc oxide cream.

- To alleviate discomfort, keep yourself and your surroundings as cool as possible. Don't take hot baths or showers. Hot water and heat brings your blood to the surface and increases the itch.

- The content of the blisters can spread the rash to other parts of your body or to other people. Cover the rash with loose, dry clothing to protect yourself and others, then handle it as little as possible. When you wash the area or apply medication, wear rubber gloves to protect your hands.

- See a doctor if you see pus or other signs of infection.

Herbal and Folk Remedies

IF YOU can locate the offending ivy/oak, look for jewelweed growing nearby. This common wildflower has a spotted orange, trumpet-shaped blossom. An ingredient in some pharmaceuticals for poison ivy, jewelweed is an excellent remedy. If you know where this plant grows and can identify it by the leaves, gather a quantity before it flowers, if possible. Puree the entire plant in an electric blender along with a little water, and smear the green paste on the rash. You can freeze the leftovers in an ice cube tray and thaw a cube when needed.

SWEET FERN, preferably gathered in November, is also said to be an effective antidote to poison ivy.

Splinters

If the splinter is visible, advises Dr. Karen Lawson, soak the area to soften and clean it, then pull out the sliver with a sterile needle or tweezers.

If the splinter is entirely under your skin, advises Dr. Lawson, apply baking soda paste or a poultice of bread soaked in milk for a couple of hours to draw the splinter to the surface. In an emergency, you could use mud for this purpose, but in urban and suburban areas mud can be contaminated with feces.

Herbal and Folk Remedies

IN THE Himalayas, latex from the fig tree is used to remove splinters and other foreign material from the skin.

Sprains

Treating sprains
Advice from Dr. Karen Lawson:

- A sprain probably won't require immediate medical attention unless a sizable bump appears within five minutes of the injury. Rapid swelling indicates bleeding and a possible broken bone. Get medical attention immediately. You could have a partially torn ligament or tendon. Resting it is protection against further damage. If you have sprained your ankle or knee, take the weight off your leg immediately.

- Ice the area to reduce pain and swelling. If you don't have crushed ice, use a bag of small or cut-up frozen vegetables for an ice pack.

- Wrap the sprain in an Ace bandage. Start from the area below your wrist or ankle and work your way up toward the knee or elbow. Be careful not to wrap so tightly that you cut off circulation. Pinch an area of exposed flesh below the bandage. If it doesn't blanch and you have no sensation, the bandage is too tight.

Herbal and Folk Remedies

••

TO EASE pain, take arnica complex, an oral homeopathic remedy, and apply an external preparation of arnica. Arnica is a mountain plant with a tiny yellow flower much esteemed in Europe, where it is used to treat sports injuries. **Warning:** Don't apply to broken skin, and don't take internally, except for oral homeopathic doses.

JUNIPER AND oregano are folk remedies for sprains. Make a strong tea, using oregano and/or juniper berries (two teaspoons to one cup boiling water), dip a cloth in the cold tea, and use as a compress to reduce pain and swelling. In a pinch, you could use a good brand of gin, which contains juniper.

A PERSIAN folk remedy is to beat one teaspoonful of turmeric into two cold egg yolks, or as many as needed to cover the sprain. Coat your wrist or ankle with the mixture, cover with gauze, then an Ace bandage, and leave on for 24 hours. Dr. Karen Lawson adds: In laboratory studies, curcuma, the active ingredient in turmeric, has been shown to reduce inflammation. Taken orally, curcuma is a better pain reliever than aspirin or other nonsteroid anti-inflammatory drugs. The oral dose is 250 milligrams curcuma and 250 milligrams slaked lime three times a day, and 500 milligrams bromelin (the active ingredient in pineapple) between meals. If you don't mind the mess, you could mix turmeric with equal parts of slaked lime and use it as a poultice for sprains. The lime is sold in health food stores and herb shops.

Sunburn

Aloe vera gel, preferably from a live plant, is very soothing and may prevent peeling. To obtain the gel, simply slit an aloe leaf lengthwise and gently scrape out the pulp with the edge of a spoon. Refrigerate any surplus for future use.

Strong tea is an Irish remedy. Steep two or three teaspoons or tea bags in a cup of boiling water for ten minutes and apply with cotton. The tannic acid, an ingredient in some pharmaceutical sunburn remedies, forms a protective surface over the burn and encourages healing.

Soak in a lukewarm bath with baking soda or oatmeal added.

Dermatologist Dr. Robin Ashinoff recommends a splash of cold milk to cool and soothe the area and aspirin or Motrin to reduce inflammation. Dr. Karen Lawson advises splashing on vinegar. Applications of cold yogurt or slices of cucumber or raw potato are also soothing.

Kitchen Cures for Common Emergencies

NOT ALL of us have a first-aid kit on hand for medical emergencies. Possibly your grandmother didn't, either. Instead, she may have headed for the pantry. Below is a list of medical applications for familiar culinary ingredients. **Note:** When making herb teas, use about a teaspoon of the dried herb or spice or two teaspoons of the fresh herb to a cup of boiling water. Boil roots and seeds or steep leaves for about ten minutes.

ALLSPICE Like most spices, allspice relieves flatulence, and like most culinary herbs, it relieves indigestion. In the Caribbean it is used internally to treat colds and flu and externally to relieve pain.

ALOE VERA Everyone should have this plant growing on a kitchen windowsill. Native Americans called it "medicine plant." So various and effective are the uses of aloe, it has been the subject of numerous laboratory studies. Most large supermarkets sell small aloe plants for a few dollars. Once you have slit one of the leaves and applied the gel to any sort of burn, including sunburn, you will consider your money well spent. The soothing gel relieves pain immediately. In tropical areas where it grows plentifully, it is used externally for headache; a teaspoon or two taken internally is gently laxative. Because it is antibacterial, the gel can also be used as a deodorant. A fungicide, it can also be diluted with 50 percent water and used to treat yeast infections and athlete's foot. Care of this succulent is easy. Plant it in cactus soil, be sure it gets lots of sun, and water only when the soil is dry.

ANISE Anise seeds are still used in folk medicine to ease cramps, gas and flatulence, indigestion, and insomnia and to stimulate milk flow in breast-feeding mothers.

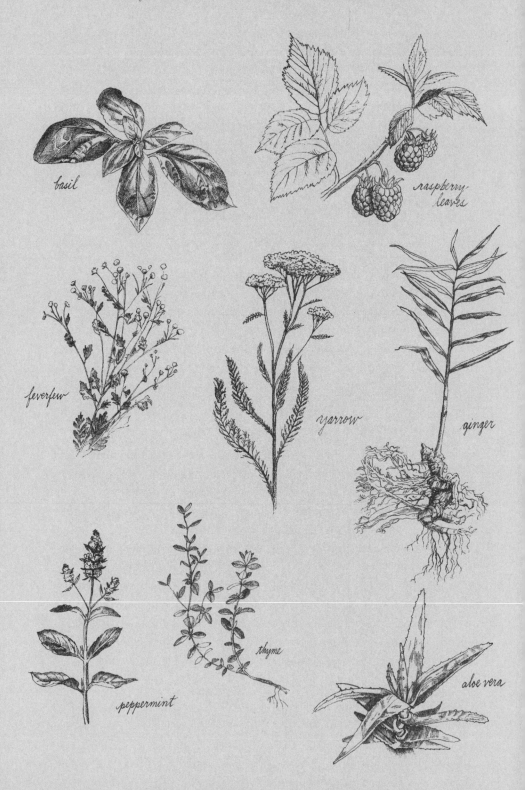

basil

raspberry leaves

feverfew

yarrow

ginger

peppermint

thyme

aloe vera

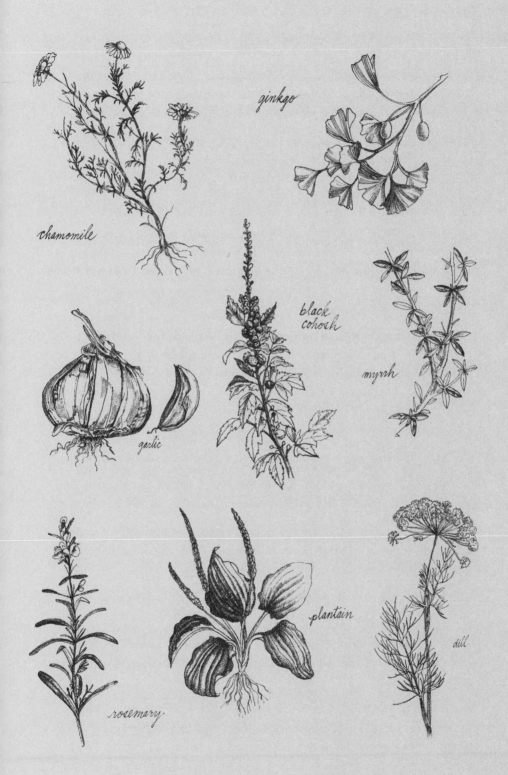

ginkgo

chamomile

black cohosh

myrrh

garlic

rosemary

plantain

dill

BAKING SODA A long-standing household remedy for skin itch and irritation. Add $1/2$ cup to a lukewarm bath to soothe sunburn and poison ivy and other skin rashes. Apply a baking-soda paste to mosquito bites and beestings and to draw out a splinter when it is under the skin. A teaspoonful in a glass of water is a traditional home remedy for gas.

BANANA To stop bleeding, mash an ordinary green banana and apply to the wound. Ripe banana arrests diarrhea.

BASIL A Romany (Gypsy) cold cure. Sip a cup of basil tea at the first sign of a sniffle.

BREAD, SPAGHETTI, ETC. Can't sleep? High-carbohydrate foods relieve tension. Eat some at bedtime if you have insomnia. Dry bread (a good homemade rye is the best kind to use) applied to a cut or wound helps draw infection; bread soaked in milk draws and dries boils and blisters.

CAYENNE PEPPER A pinch or two of this tropical pepper in your food or drink stimulates circulation and perspiration and warms you up. For a quick liniment or pain reliever, add about $1/4$ teaspoon to a cup of alcohol or oil and massage your aching joints or muscles with it. Sprinkle some in your socks to warm your feet. At the first sign of a cold, add liberally to your food and sprinkle a pinch or two on a cup of hot water with a tablespoon each of cider vinegar and honey.

CINNAMON Sip a cup of cinnamon tea for indigestion and flatulence.

CLOVES Got a toothache? Put a few drops of cloves oil in the cavity for immediate relief. Drink clove tea to prevent vomiting and relieve nausea.

COFFEE Three cups of lukewarm or cool coffee can head off an asthma attack: the caffeine is a potent bronchodilator. Caffeinated tea will also work, but you need to drink six cups.

DILL Since antiquity, the seeds of this delicious herb has been used to treat colic, insomnia, and tension, and to promote the flow of breast milk.

FENNEL Tea made from these licorice-flavored seeds is excellent for relieving gas. A compress made from the seeds soothes eyestrain and eye irritation.

FROZEN VEGETABLES Crushed ice applied externally is a painkiller *par excellence,* but not an item most of us have on hand unless we are giving a party. A bag of frozen peas, corn, carrots, or other small or cut-up vegetables makes a perfect ice pack. Apply it to sprained wrists and ankles, bumps and swellings, arthritis and other inflammations, black eyes, bee stings, and insect bites. Some headaches yield miraculously to an ice pack applied to the back of the neck. Ice stops bleeding and ice water soothes burns. Don't apply the ice directly to your skin, however—wrap it in a towel or cloth, and don't leave it on for longer than ten minutes at a time.

GARLIC If you expect to be stranded on a desert island, this is the herb to take along. Recorded medicinal uses of garlic date back to ancient Egypt; they are so numerous it would almost be easier to list instances where you don't use garlic. Rub a cut raw clove over a beesting to relieve irritation. Tuck a raw clove in your cheek when you feel a cold coming on; chop a raw clove fine and add a tablespoon of honey for coughs and congestion. The hardworking garlic clove, taken internally, is also recommended for both diarrhea and constipation. Unpeeled, it can be used as a suppository for hemorrhoids; peeled (be careful not to nick it), as a suppository for vaginal infections.

GIN Take a shot or two to relieve menstrual cramps. Chill and use as a compress for sprains. **Warning:** Don't use when pregnant.

GINGER Like garlic, ginger has a long history of universal usage. In Chinese medicine it is considered a warming herb and used in tea to ward off a cold. It has also been shown to be as effective as Dramamine at relieving motion sickness. For nausea, boil about three slices of fresh root or infuse a teaspoon of powdered ginger and sip the tea. Ginger is antibiotic and has been used to treat salmonella. More recently, the root has been shown to prevent blood platelets from sticking together, suggesting its efficacy in treating rheumatism and respiratory problems and stimulating circulation.

HONEY When you have insomnia, add a tablespoonful of honey to hot milk along with a dash of nutmeg. To ward off a cold, dissolve two tablespoons each honey and cider vinegar in a cup of hot water, add a pinch of cayenne pepper, and drink hot at bedtime. For constipation, drink a glass of hot water with a tablespoon of honey dissolved in it. If you burn yourself with hot cooking oil, apply honey.

LEMON JUICE An infection fighter. Put a few drops in your ear when you have an earache; dilute slightly and use as a wash for cuts and wounds. To ease constipation, drink the juice of one lemon in a cup of hot water before breakfast.

MARJORAM A member of the mint family, marjoram has medicinal uses similar to those for mint. Infuse the leaves for headache, tension, indigestion, gas and flatulence, and respiratory problems. The oil dulls the pain of an aching tooth and of muscular aches and stiffness.

MEAT TENDERIZER Sprinkle some on bee stings—papain, the active ingredient, digests the protein in the bee venom.

MINT The uses are similar to those for marjoram. The tea soothes menstrual cramps and stomachache. To break up nasal congestion, add a handful of peppermint to a bowl of hot water and lean over the bowl with a towel draped over your head. Don't get too close to the water—steam can burn!

MUSTARD Until recent decades, powdered mustard seeds were the basis of at least four popular home remedies: **mustard plaster,** applied to the chest to relieve bronchial congestion (equal parts mustard, flour, and tepid water); **mustard poultice,** applied to stiff, sore muscles to ease aches and pains ($3/4$ cup linseed meal, $1/3$ cup mustard, one cup boiling water); **mustard footbath,** an old-fashioned cold preventative (a tablespoon of mustard to each gallon of hot water); and an **emetic** to induce vomiting (one teaspoon mustard to a glass of warm water).

NUTMEG Like other culinary spices, nutmeg relieves gas and indigestion. When you feel tense and sleepless, sip a cup of hot milk with $1/2$ teaspoon nutmeg and a tablespoon honey added.

OATMEAL Soothes skin irritation. Apply as a paste to soothe and dry poison oak and ivy blisters.

OLIVE OIL Apply to burns; swallow a tablespoonful for constipation.

ONION For infected cuts, wounds, and abrasions, squeeze or mash a raw onion to express the juice. Apply the juice after you have washed the infected area with soap and water.

AN OLD folk remedy for earache: bake an onion until soft, apply to your aching ear, cover with a cloth or bandage, and attach with tape.

PAPAYA Mash the pulp and use it to stop bleeding, or apply to bee sting. The pulp is laxative.

ROSEMARY This fragrant herb has a centuries-old reputation for stimulating the circulation and soothing aches and pains. For quick relief of strained muscles or arthritic joints, gently heat about $\frac{1}{4}$ cup rosemary in a cup of olive or vegetable oil for about a half hour. Use as a massage oil while still warm. Leftover oil can be rewarmed in a glass container set in a saucepan of simmering water.

TEA The tannin in tea soothes sunburn. Brew a strong cup—a tablespoon steeped in a cup of boiling water for ten minutes; cool, and apply with cotton. Apply a wet tea bag to take the sting from a fever blister or to relieve sore nipples. In a pinch, caffeinated tea may head off an asthma attack, but you have to drink a lot—six cups.

THYME Use the oil, mixed with water, as a wash for wounds. Thyme oil is antiseptic and was once used in hospitals as a disinfectant.

TURMERIC The active ingredient is curcuma, which in laboratory studies has proved more effective than aspirin and other non-steroidal anti-inflammatory pain relievers. Use it in a poultice for inflammation, or drink tea made with it.

VINEGAR Splash on burns and sunburn. Apply to wasp stings.

RESOURCES

For more information about a specific ailment, contact one of the following organizations. Some also make referrals to physicians in your area who specialize in treating your particular health problem.

Organizations

Allen and Hanbury's Respiratory Institute, 5 Moore Drive, Research Triangle Park, NC 27709. Call 1-800-843-2474 to receive educational material on respiratory diseases, for a free subscription to *Air Currents,* an eight-page quarterly newsletter, or information about recycling medication containers.

Alternative Health Insurance Services. Call 1-800-331-2713 for names of health insurers who cover alternative medical care.

American Academy of Dermatology, P.O. Box 681069, Schamburg, IL 60168. They offer fifty different pamphlets, continuously updated, about skin problems. To receive one or more, send a stamped, self-addressed legal-size envelope to the above address. For local, nationwide, or international physician referrals only call 1-708-330-0230.

American Academy of Otolaryngology—Head and Neck Surgery, 1 Prince Street, Alexandria, VA 22314. Send stamped, self-addressed envelope for a list of brochures on ear and throat disorders.

American Allergy Association, P.O. Box 640, Menlo Park, CA 94026. Call 1-415-322-1663 for catalog or information about publications.

American Association of Naturopathic Physicians, 2366 Eastlake Avenue East, Suite 322, Seattle, WA 98102. Send $5.00 for national directory of naturopathic physicians and information about naturopathy.

American Botanical Council, P.O. Box 201660, Austin, TX 78720. Disseminates information about herbs and medicinal plants, publishes *Herbalgram,* a quarterly detailing current research on medicinal herbs. To receive 20-page catalog or *Herbalgram* ($25.00/year), call 1-800-373-7105.

American Center for the Alexander Technique, 129 West 67th Street, New York, NY 10023. 1-212-799-0468.

American Chronic Pain Association, P.O. Box 850, Rocklin, CA 95677. Offers training in coping with pain; helps you locate pain unit, has support groups. Call 1-800-444-8991 to receive packet of information about chronic pain.

American Council for Headache Education, 875 Kings Highway, Suite 200, West Deptford, NJ 08094. Call 1-800-255-2243 for information about support groups, referrals to health practitioners in your area who treat headache, or educational literature pertaining to headache.

American Heart Association, 7320 Greenville Avenue, Dallas, TX 75231. 1-800-AHA-USA1 (1-800-242-8721).

American Herbalists Guild, P.O. Box 1683, Soquel, CA 95073. 1-408-464-2441.

American Holistic Medical Association, 4101 Lake Boone Trail, Suite 201, Raleigh, NC 27607. 1-919-787-5181.

The American Institute of Stress, 124 Park Avenue, Yonkers, NY 10703. Monthly newsletter reports on current stress research $35.00/year; general information packet on stress $25.00; specific topics $35.00 for 15–20 pages.

American Lung Association. To connect with your local chapter, call 800-LUNG-USA.

American Sleep Disorders Association, 604 2nd Street SW, Rochester, MN 55902. Write them for general information and list of sleep labs nationwide.

Aradia Feminist Women's Health Center 1300 Spring Street, Seattle, WA 98104. 1-205-323-9388

The Arthritis Foundation. Call 1-800-283-7800 for literature; leave your name and address. Your local chapter will send literature about arthritis.

Boston Women's Health Collective, Box 192, West Somerville, MA 02144. 1-617-625-0271; fax: 1-617-625-0294. Research, referrals, information; library open to the public. Advocates for women's health, authored *Our Bodies, Ourselves* and *The New Our Bodies, Ourselves.*

Center for Science in the Public Interest, 1875 Connecticut Avenue NW, Suite 300, Washington, DC 20009-5728. Advocate for improved health and nutrition policies, informative newsletter.

Fibromyalgia Network, P.O. Box 31750, Tucson, AZ 85751-1750.

Homeopathic Educational Services, 2124 Kittredge Street, Berkeley CA 94704. Educational materials, directory of homeopathic practitioners.

Hysterectomy Educational Resources and Services Foundation, 422 Bryn Mawr Avenue, Bala Cynwyd, PA 19004. 1-610-667-7757. Educational literature, free phone counseling.

National Association of People with AIDS, 1413 K Street NW, Washington, DC 20005. 1-202-898-0414; fax: 1-202-898-0435. Information, referrals, list of educational literature.

National Asthma and Allergy Network, 10875 Main Street, Suite 210, Fairfax, VA 22030. 1-703-385-4403.

National Heart, Lung and Blood Institute. Free 60-page reading and resource list available from its National Asthma Education Program, NHBLI Information Center, P.O. Box 30105, Bethesda, MD 20824-0105. 1-301-951-3260.

National Osteoporosis Foundation— National Headquarters 1-202-223-2226.

North American Society of Teachers of the Alexander Technique, Box 806, Ansonia Station, New York, NY 10023. 1-800-473-0620. Maintains list of certified teacher members.

Office of Disease Prevention & Health Promotions' National Center for Health Information, P.O. Box 1133, Washington, DC 20013-1133, 1-800-336-4797. Call or write for list of toll-free numbers of federal health information centers and clearinghouses.

PMS Treatment Center, Department SF, P.O. Box 20998, Portland, OR 97220. Send stamped, self-addressed envelope, $5.00, and state you are interested in for list of health professionals in your area who treat PMS.

Vestibular Disorders Association, 1015 NW 22nd Avenue, D—230, Portland, OR. 1-800-837-8428. Literature and information on inner-ear disorders.

Newsletters

Air Currents. Free 8-page bimonthly newsletter on asthma. Free from Allen and Hanbury's Respiratory Institute, 5 Moore Drive, Research Triangle Park, NC 27709. 1-800-843-2474.

Asthma Update Newsletter for People with Asthma, 123 Monticello Avenue, Annapolis, MD 21401. 410-267-8329. $10.00/year; send stamped, self-addressed envelope for free sample.

Harvard Women's Health Watch, 164 Longwood Avenue, Boston, MA 02115. 1-617-432-1485. Reports on women's health research. $24.00/year; single copies $4.00.

Healthfacts, monthly, with $21.00 membership in Center for Medical Consumers, 237 Thompson Street, New York, NY 10012.

Nutrition Action. Published by Center for Science in the Public Interest, 1875 Connecticut Avenue NW, Suite 300, Washington, DC 20009-5728. $24.00/year. Current updates on nutrition research.

The Townsend Letter, 911 Tyler St., Port Townsend, WA 98368, 1-206-385-6021. $42.00/year (10 issues). Directed to homeopathic and naturopathic physicians.

Libraries and Research Services

Boston Women's Health Collective, 240A Elm Street, West Somerville, MA. 1-617-625-0271. Files and publications devoted to women's health issues. Call for hours.

Center for Medical Consumers, 237 Thompson Street, New York, NY 10012. 1-212-674-7105. Books, medical journals and other publications, extensive files on traditional and alternative therapies for a wide variety of disorders.

The Health Resource, 564 Locust Street, Conway, AR 72032. 1-800-949-0090. Reports, referrals, newsletter. Reports are at least 50 pages; most are 195–295 pages.

The Lloyd Library, 917 Plum Street, Cincinnati, OH. 1-513-721-3707. Fax: 1-513-721-6575. E-mail: Michael Flannery at UC.EDU. Specializes in botanical pharmacology, answers questions. Over 200,000 books, 600 journals cover Western, Chinese, Ayurvedic, and other pharmacologies. Historical collection goes back to 1493.

Lung Facts. Automated information service with recorded messages on 77 topics, sponsored by the National Jewish Center. During business hours you can speak with a nurse. Call 1-800-522-LUNG.

National Cancer Institute. By calling 1-800-4-CANCER, you can get a free printout from its database on state-of-the-art treatment of specific forms of cancer, and referrals to community resources.

World Research Foundation, 15300 Ventura Boulevard, Suite 405, Sherman Oaks, CA 91403. 1-800-WRF-HELP; in California, call 1-818-907-5483. Computer and library searches, bibliographies. Provides information on both conventional and alternative therapies for most major health concerns. Computer searches run to 50 pages; packets of library material, up to 500 pages. Average search costs about $45.00, plus tax and shipping. Library open to the public.

Mail Order Sources for Herbs

Aphrodisia, 264 Bleeker Street, New York, NY 10014. 1-212-989-6440. Wide variety of medicinal herbs, some organic, also Chinese and Ayurvedic botanicals, ginseng, and homeopathic remedies.

Caprilands Herb Farm, 534 Silver Street, Coventry, CT 06238. 1-203-742-7244. Dried medicinal and culinary herbs, also seeds and live plants. Extensive gardens, great place to visit, superb herbal luncheons.

Indiana Botanic Gardens, Inc., Box 5, Hammond, IN 46325. 1-800-644-8327. One of the oldest and best. Wide assortment of single herbs and mixtures based on early American and European spa recipes; excellent book list.

BIBLIOGRAPHY

Abraham, Guy E., M.D., and Harinder Grewel, M.D. "A Total Dietary Program Emphasizing Magnesium Instead of Calcium." *Journal of Reproductive Medicine.*

American Academy of Dermatology. "Animal Studies Suggest Skin Aging Can be Reversed" and "For Women with Facial Pigmentation, Try Peeling It Away" (press releases).

American Academy of Ophthalmology. "Cataract Surgery," "Dry Eye," "Contact Lenses and Cosmetics," "Glaucoma," "Floaters and Flashers," "Chalazion," "Blepharitis," "Macular Degeneration and Nutrition," and "Sunglasses" (information sheets).

American Academy of Otolaryngology. "Swimmers' Ear," "Ears, Altitude and Airplane Travel," "Dizziness and Motion Sickness," "Earwax," "Nose Bleeds," "Clearing the Air," "Your Nose Knows," and "You and Your Stuffy Nose" (information sheets).

American Chronic Pain Association. "Ten Concepts—Moving from Patient to Person" (leaflet).

American College of Rheumatology. "Reporters Guide to Arthritis" (booklet).

American Council for Headache Education. "Stress and Headache" (report).

American Heart Association. "Silent Epidemic: The Truth About Women and Heart Disease" (leaflet).

American Lung Association. "Common Cold," "Influenza," "Pneumonia," "Chronic Bronchitis," "Second Hand Smoke," "Nicotine Addiction and Cigarettes," "Cigarette Smoking," "Asthma," "Home Control of Allergies and Asthma," "The Asthma Handbook," and "Help Yourself to Better Breathing" (leaflets).

American Medical Association. *AMA Pocket Guide to Sports First Aid.* New York: Random House, 1993.

Anderson, Bob. *Stretching.* Bolinas, Calif.: Shelter Publications, 1980.

Annals of Internal Medicine. Reports on evening primrose oil for arthritis. (November 1, 1995, and January 1994).

Aquavella, Dr. James V.; Dr. Herbert E. Kaufman; and Dr. R. D. Richards. Article on avoiding and treating eye infections. *Patient Care* (September 1988).

Arthritis Foundation. "Exercise and Your Arthritis" (pamphlet).

Asthma Update Newsletter. 10:1 (Summer 1994); 9:4 (Spring 1994).

Bethel, May. *The Healing Power of Herbs.* London: Thorsons Publishers, 1968.

Britt, Jennifer, and Lesley Keen. *Feverfew.* London: Century Hutchinson, 1987.

Brody, David M., M.D. "Running Injuries." *Clinical Symposia* 39:3 (March 1987).

Brown, Donald J., N. D. "Alternative Approaches to Tinnitus, Menière's Disease and Hearing Loss." *Let's Live* (October 1993).

Burros, Marian. "Some Wives' Tales Withstand Scrutiny." *The New York Times*, February 23, 1994.

Bush, Dr. A. D. *Potters Compendium of Materia Medica Therapeutics and Prescription Writing*. Philadelphia: P. Blakiston's Son and Co., 1917.

Carper, Jean. *The Food Pharmacy*. New York: Bantam Books, 1988.

Center for Science in the Public Interest. Report on cataracts. Newsletter, January/February 1991.

Clark, Roland, M.D.; Joseph M. Farber, M.D.; and Neal Sher, M.D. Article on eye emergencies. *Patient Care*, January 15, 1989.

Consumer Reports. "Alternative Medicine: The Facts." January 1994.

Fatemi, Shireen; Elizabeth Ryzen; Jose Flores; David B. Endres; and Robert K. Rude. "Effect of Experimental Human Magnesium Depletion on Parathyroid Hormone Secretion and 1,25 Dihydroxy Vitamin D Metabolism." *Journal of Clinical Endocrinology and Metabolism* 73:5.

Fishbein, Morris, M.D. *The Handy Home Medical Adviser and Concise Medical Encyclopedia*. Garden City, N.Y.: Doubleday and Company, 1963.

Forstall, Gregory J., M.D.; Michael L. Macknin, M.D.; Belinda R. Yen-Lieberman, Ph.D.; and Sharon Vanderbrug Mendendorp, M.P.H. "Effects of Inhaling Heated Vapor on Symptoms of the Common Cold." *Journal of the American Medical Association* 27:14 (April 13, 1994).

Frawley, Dr. David, and Dr. Vasant Lad. *The Yoga of Herbs*. Santa Fe: Lotus Press, 1986.

Freeman, Sally. *Herbs for All Seasons*. New York: New American Library/Plume, 1991.

————. *The Green World*. New York: Berkeley, 1975.

Gardner, Joy. "Healing Your Family's Colds." *Mothering*, Winter 1990.

Gibbons, Euell. *Stalking the Wild Asparagus*. New York: David McKay Company, 1970.

Hamburg, Joan F. "Can Home Remedies Work?" *Parade*, July 31, 1994.

Harvard Women's Health Letter. Report on caffeine and sleep, April 1994; report on chicken collagen for rheumatoid arthritis, January 1994.

Healey, Father Joseph G., and Donald F. Syberty. *I Pointed Out the Stars*. Orvis Books, 1993.

Heart, Lung, and Blood Institute. "Teach Your Patients About Asthma" and "Management of Asthma During Pregnancy."

Hendley, J. Owen, M.D.; Robert D. Abbott, Ph.D.; Patsy P. Beasley, R.N.; and Jack M. Gwaltney, Jr., M.D. "Effect of Inhalation of Hot Humidified Air on Experimental Rhinovirus Infection." *Journal of the American Medical Association* 271:14 (April 13, 1994).

Herb Research Foundation and American Botanical Council. *Herbal Gram* 16, 18, 19, 21, 22, 25, 26, and 30.

Hoffman, David. *The New Holistic Herbal*. Rockport, Mass.: Element, Inc., 1992.

Kent, Carol Miller. *Aloe Vera*. Arlington, Va.: Carol Miller Kent, 1979.

Kloss, Jethro. *Back to Eden*. New York: Benedict Lust Publications, 1971.

Kolata, Gina. "In Ancient Times, Flowers and Fennel for Family Planning." *The New York Times*, March 8, 1994.

Kordel, Lelord. *Natural Folk Remedies*. New York: G. P. Putnam's Sons, 1974.

Lancet, The. Report on Norwegian study on rheumatoid arthritis and fasting (1991); Letter on using powdered vitamin C as snuff for colds (November 1989).

Lane, Hilary. "Sip by Sipping in the 90's." *Food and Heatlh*, September/October 1993.

Leary, Warren E. "2 Healthful Bacteria Are Proved to Ward Off Diarrhea in Infants." *The New York Times*, October 14, 1994.

Lee, John, M.D. "Significance of Molecular Configuration Specificity—The Case of Progesterone and Osteoporosis." *Townsend Letter for Doctors*, June 1993. "Osteoporosis Reversal." *International Clinical Nutrition Review*, June 1990.

Lucas, Richard. *Nature's Medicines*. New York: Award Books, 1969.

Lust, John. *The Herb Book*. New York: Benedict Lust Publications, 1974.

McNeill, F. Marian. *Recipes from Scotland*. Albyn Press, 1946.

Makgoba, M. W., and H. K. Datta. "The Critical Role of Magnesium Ions in Osteoclastmatrix Interaction." *European Journal of Clinical Investigation* 22 (1992): 692–96.

Medical SelfCare. Report on headaches. November 12, 1989.

Modern Medicine. Report on itchy ears. August 1988. Article on anemia. August 1992.

Moyers, Bill. *Healing and the Mind*. New York: Doubleday, a division of Bantam Doubleday Dell, 1993.

Murray, Michael, N.D., and Joseph Pizzorno, N.D., *Encyclopedia of Natural Medicine*. Rocklin, Calif.: Prima Publishing, 1991.

Nagarathna R., and Nagendra, H.R., "Yoga for Bronchial Asthma: A Controlled Study." *British Medical Journal* 291 (October 19, 1985).

National Dairy Council. "Fat Information Sheet," "Cholesterol Information Sheet," and "Calcium Information Sheet." 1981.

National Sleep Foundation. "The Nature of Sleep and Its Disorders" (pamphlet).

Natural Health Magazine. "Bodywork" column: "Feeling Down." November/December 1993.

New Scientist. Report on sleep: current research. November 13, 1993.

Nielsen, Forrest H. "Studies on the Relationship Between Boron and Magnesium Which Possibly Affects Formation and Maintenance of Bones." Paper delivered by author at Fifth Annual Meeting of American Society for Magnesium Research, September 26, 1989.

Nobel, Elizabeth. *Essential Exercises for the Childbearing Years*.

Ody, Penelope. *The Complete Medicinal Herbal*. London: Dorling Kindersley, 1993.

Panos, Maesimund B., M.D., and Jane Heimlich. *Homeopathic Medicine*. Los Angeles: J. P. Archer, 1980.

Parker, Karen. Article on anemia in pregnancy. *Birthing*, January 1985.

Patient Care. Article on colds. January 15, 1990. Article on vertigo and ear infections. September 30, 1990.

The Physical Medicine and Rehabilitation Center, Pa. "Sprains, Strains and Tears," "Tennis Elbow," "Osteoarthritis," "Myofacial Pain Syndrome," "Osteoporosis," "Discogenic Low Back Pain," and "Managing Chronic Pain" (pamphlets).

Reitz, Rosetta. *Menopause: A Positive Approach*. New York: Penguin Books, 1977.

Rinzler, Carol Ann. *Feed a Cold, Starve a Fever*. New York: Ballantine Books, 1979, 1991. (Originally *The Dictionary of Medical Folklore* [New York: Thomas Y. Crowell, 1979].)

Rodale Press Editors. *The Illustrated Encyclopedia of Herbs*. Emmaus, Pa.: Rodale Press, 1987; "The Good Fats." Emmaus, Pa.: Rodale Press, 1988 (booklet).

Rosenberg, Dr. Robert. "Lighting and the Aging Eye." *Aging and Vision News*, Winter/Spring 1994.

Science News. Report on immunity and aspirin. May 1989.

Seligson, Susan V. Report on dry eyes. *Health*, March/April 1991.

Shangold, Mona, M.D., and Gabe Mirkin, M.D. *The Complete Sports Medicine Book for Women*. New York: Simon and Schuster, 1985.

Shastri, Vijay. *Journal of Scientific Research in Plants and Medicines*. Hardwar, India: Yogi Pharmacy.

Siegal, Karen H. "The Alexander Technique." *Behavioral Medicine*, November/December 1981.

Simmonite, Dr. W. J., and Nicholas Culpeper. *Herbal Remedies*. New York: Award Books/London: Tandem Books, 1957.

Talbert, Lee, and Michelle M. Pauly. "Bilberry" (pamphlet).

Toomay, Mindy. *A Cozy Book of Herbal Teas*. Rocklin, Calif.: Prima Publishing, 1994.

Tyler, Varro. *The New Honest Herbal*. Philadelphia, George F. Stickley, 1987.

Vestibular Disorders Association. "Earache and Otis Media" and "Ears, Altitude and Airplane Travel" (leaflets).

Von Hausen, Wanja. *Gypsy Folk Medicine*. New York: Sterling Publishing Co., 1992.

Washburn, Kenneth B., M.D., and Murray A. Swanson. *Neck Care*. Redmond, Wash.: Medic Publishing Co., 1979 (booklet).

Weil, Andrew, M.D. *Natural Health, Natural Medicine*. Boston: Houghton Mifflin, 1960.

Weiss, Rudolph Fritz. *Herbal Medicine*. Gothenburg, Germany: Arcanum, 1988.

West Virginia Medical Journal. Report on allergy and Menière's syndrome. September 1974.

White, Isabella Maxwell. *The Scottish Bakehouse Cook Book*. Tashmoo Press, 1972.

Whitlock, Evelyn P., M.D. *The Calcium Plus Workbook*. New Canaan, Conn.: Keats Publishing, 1988.

Wilford, John Noble. "Ancient Tree Yields Secrets of Potent Healing Substance." *The New York Times*, March 1, 1988.

World Mission. Report on African folk medicine. March 1994.

Index

Epsom salts, 25, 58, 88, 124, 195
Equalactin, 61
Ergot, 15, 221
Estradiol, 22
Estrogen, 22–23, 26
Estrone, 22
Eucalyptus, 104, 209, 224
Eustachian tube, 174
Evening primrose oil, 125
Excessive menstruation, 29–30
Exercise, 45, 73, 80, 121, 140–141, 146, 156
Expectorant, 7
Eye infections, 185
Eye injuries, 226–227
Eye problems, 181–192
Eyebright, 184, 186
Eyes, 181
  bags under, 181
  black, 182, 219–220
  bloodshot, 182
  chemicals in, 226
  cinder or other foreign material in, 226–227
  dry, 186–187
  hit by object in, 227
  irritated, 189
  itchy, 189
  puffy, 191
Eyestrain, 188–189

F
Fainting, 227–228
False labor, 14–15
Fatigue, 159–160
Fats, 79
Feet
  athlete's, 197
  and hands, cold, 81–83
  and legs in pregnancy, swelling of, 17
  problems with, 133–134
Fennel, 12, 184, 186, 236
Fenugreek, 48, 52
Fertility cycle, 18
Fever, 109
Feverfew, 123, 164, 208, 212, 234
Fiber, 45
Fibrocystic breasts, 21
Fibroids, uterine, 21

Fibromyalgia, 134–135
Flatulence, 53–54
Floaters in vision field, 192
Flu, 100–104
Fo-ti, 23, 160
Folic acid, 18, 33
Folk medicine, 7
Folk remedies, 2–3
Food diary, 53
Foot, *see* Feet
Freckles, 196
Frozen vegetables, 236–237

G
Gargling, 115, 116
Garlic, 39, 50, 60, 64, 80–81, 85, 98, 101, 105, 106, 133, 196, 217, 219, 235, 237
Gas, 53–54
Gin, 237
Ginger, 34, 48, 54, 57, 67, 68, 80, 82, 101, 107, 234, 237
Gingivitis, 63
Ginkgo, 81, 99, 159, 181, 235
Ginseng, 23, 36, 101
Glare, preventing, 188–189
Glossary, 5–8
Gloves, 82
Glucosamine sulfate, 123
Gluten, 61
Glycerin, 201
Goldenseal, 13, 50, 65, 67, 176, 186, 195, 208, 224
Goldthread, 65
Gotu kola, 160, 208, 212
Gums, bleeding, 63–64

H
Hair, 194
  dry, 202–203
  dull, 205–206
  thinning, 213–214
Hamstring injury, 149–150
Hand lotion, 205
Hands and feet, cold, 81–83
Hangover, 55
Hawthorn, 81, 85, 87, 89
Hay fever, 112–113
HDL (high-density lipoprotein), 79, 80
Headache, 161–164

Weight management, 73–74
Weightlifting tips, 141–142
Windburn, 201
Wine, 80
Wintergreen, 124
Witch hazel, 58–59, 91, 198, 219
Work stations, 142–143
Worms, 59–60
Wormwood, 60
Wounds, 223–225
Woundwort, 224
Wrinkles, 205

Y
Yarrow, 30, 175, 224, 234
Yeast infections, 41–42
Yerba santa, 105
Yerbabuena, 52, 105, 157
Yoga, 27, 35, 63, 73
Yogurt, 49
Yogurt douche, 40

Z
Zinc, 32, 219
Zostrix, 213

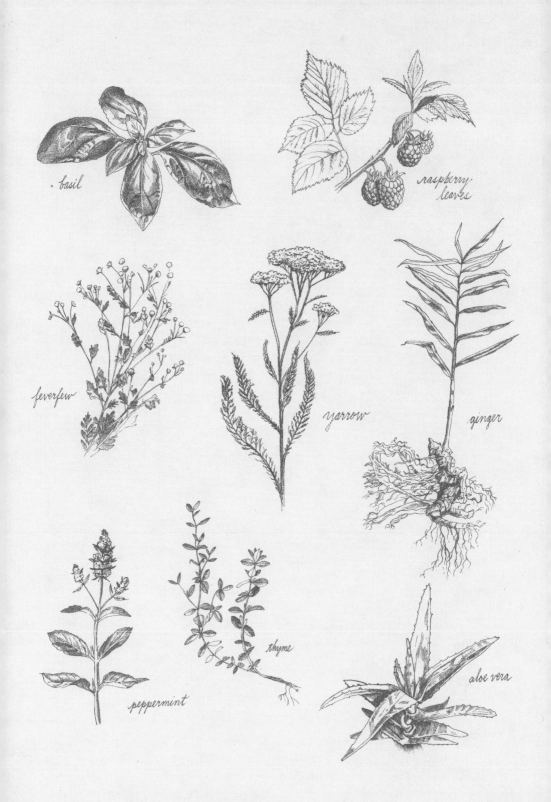

basil

raspberry leaves

feverfew

yarrow

ginger

peppermint

thyme

aloe vera